THE HOLISTIC ROOT TO MANAGING ANXIETY

HEALING FROM THE INSIDE OUT

SECOND EDITION

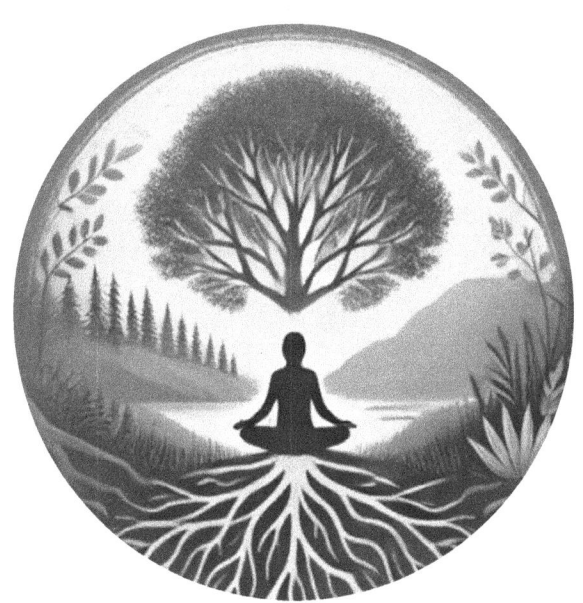

Maria Tabone, MS, MA, CNS

The Holistic Root to Managing Anxiety:
Healing Anxiety from the Inside Out

Copyright © 2025 by Maria Tabone, MS, MA, CNS

www.theholisticroot.com

Email: maria@theholisticroot.com

Published by Maria Tabone, Summit, NJ

All rights reserved. No part of this book may be reproduced, other than for "fair use" as brief quotations embodied in articles and reviews, without prior written permission from the publisher.

About the Author

Maria Tabone is an Integrative Nutritionist, Duke Trained and Certified Health & Well-Being Coach / National Board-Certified Health & Well-Being Coach (NBHWC), Certified Functional Nutrition Coach, Certified Ayurveda Practitioner, Herbalist (AHG) and Clinical Aromatherapist. She is also a Registered Yoga & Meditation Teacher, Educator, Speaker, and Author with over 20 years of experience in the integrative health field.

Maria holds two Master's degrees, one in Integrative Health & Healing and another in Health & Nutrition Education, along with a certification in Plant-Based Nutrition from Cornell University. She also has advanced training in Reflexology, Reiki, Chakra Balancing, and other holistic modalities.

Her passion for integrative healing began with her own health challenges which inspired her to seek natural solutions when conventional medicine fell short. Today she blends ancient wisdom with modern science to help women heal through a personalized, lifestyle-based approach. Her areas of focus include weight loss, thyroid disease, chronic illness, and anxiety.

Maria is the author of The Holistic Root to Managing Anxiety: Healing from the Inside Out and co-host of the podcast Unpacking Midlife with the Wise Women, available on Apple and Spotify.

She specializes in nutrition and wellness consulting for many conditions, including anxiety, depression, autoimmune disease, high cholesterol, metabolic syndrome, thyroid disease, and weight management.

Contact information: maria@theholisticroot.com

To my husband Vincent who supports me in everything I do.

To all who live with anxiety—

May this book remind you that healing is possible,

that your story matters,

and that you are never alone on this journey.

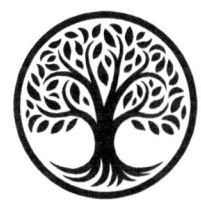

Contents

Preface to the Second Edition ix

CHAPTER 1 What is Anxiety? 1

CHAPTER 2 Social Media and the Pace of Modern Life 6

CHAPTER 3 Acupuncture 10

CHAPTER 4 Aromatherapy 12

CHAPTER 5 Ayurveda 20

CHAPTER 6 Bach Flower Essences 26

CHAPTER 7 Bodywork 30

CHAPTER 8 Breathing 33

CHAPTER 9 CBD aka Cannabidiol 36

CHAPTER 10 Diet 43

CHAPTER 11 Digestive Health 48

CHAPTER 12 Emotional Freedom Technique 52

CHAPTER	13	Exercise	59
CHAPTER	14	Herbs	63
CHAPTER	15	Homeopathy	73
CHAPTER	16	Meditation	76
CHAPTER	17	Music Therapy	79
CHAPTER	18	Religion and Spirituality	82
CHAPTER	19	Sleep	85
CHAPTER	20	Social Connection	87
CHAPTER	21	Acceptance and Commitment Therapy (ACT)	90
CHAPTER	22	Biofeedback	94
CHAPTER	23	Cognitive Behavioral Therapy	97
CHAPTER	24	Eye Movement Desensitization and Reprocessing (EMDR)	100
CHAPTER	25	Health Coaching	104
CHAPTER	26	Therapy	108
CHAPTER	27	What's Next?	111

References	115
Resources	122

Disclaimer

The information in this book is based on the author's experience and research and has not been evaluated by the FDA. This information is not intended to treat, diagnose, cure, or prevent any disease. It is not intended as a substitute for consulting with your physician or other healthcare providers. Check with your doctor before starting any new program.

If you are experiencing severe anxiety, depression, difficulty functioning in daily life, or thoughts of self-harm, please seek immediate professional help. Reaching out for mental health support is often essential. You are not alone, and there is no shame in asking for help.

Many find relief by blending conventional and holistic methods. Licensed mental health professionals can provide crucial support in understanding and addressing the root causes of anxiety. It is highly advisable to seek guidance from a trained professional when dealing with persistent anxiety.

Additionally, if you are pregnant, please consult your healthcare provider before using any essential oils or herbal remedies.

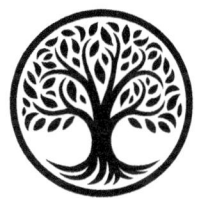

Preface to the Second Edition

Much has changed since this book's first edition over a decade ago. We experienced the COVID-19 pandemic, which has had far-reaching effects on mental health and contributed to the rising levels of anxiety worldwide. Politics has become increasingly contentious, causing rifts among family and friends. In addition, social media has introduced new complexities into our lives. While it offers convenience and connectivity, it also fuels confusion, comparison, and a constant sense of inadequacy. Unfortunately, anxiety has become an all-too-common response to the overload of external stimuli, unrealistic expectations, and the pressures of modern life. The nature of truth and facts has come under scrutiny, leaving many uncertain about what to believe, further heightening anxiety.

The combination of health fears, social isolation, economic insecurity, and uncertainty has made it increasingly difficult to navigate life's challenges. Change is a part of life, but it has become hard to manage, especially when compounded by existing stressors. This environment has created the perfect storm for anxiety to flourish. In our fast-paced, digitally distracted world, it's easy to lose connection with ourselves and ignore signs of stress until they become overwhelming. The good news is that you have the power to take control and manage your life.

I understand how anxiety can affect someone's life. When you are in the middle of those symptoms, it can be all-encompassing and incapacitating.

My personal story with anxiety began years ago when I landed a great job. Everything ran smoothly for over a year. Afterwards, my manager, a wonderful person, was succeeded by someone who was unkind, patronizing, and very demanding. What had once been a dream job turned into a nightmare.

After six months in a hostile work environment, I began experiencing bouts of vertigo, broke out in large, circular hives across my legs and stomach, and had episodes of shortness of breath. Fearing it might be heart-related, especially since my father died of a heart attack at fifty-five, I went to see my doctor.

My doctor conducted a thorough examination and said I was in perfect health. He then offered me a prescription for anti-anxiety medication, along with a referral to a neurologist. The neurologist administered a straightforward test involving touching my nose and marching in place.

Upon learning about my stressful work situation, he, too, recommended anti-anxiety medication. It felt like a quick fix: touch your nose, and here's a pill! It was not the outcome I expected.

Dissatisfied with both doctors' swift prescription approach, I made an appointment with a new primary care physician with an integrative perspective. After conducting a physical examination, he asked me about my life. I was surprised, as I had never been asked that by a doctor before. I shared that, in addition to my job stress, my mother had been diagnosed with pancreatic cancer. After listening with patience and compassion, he acknowledged that my mother was nearing the end of her life. He suggested that after she passed, I return in about six months for another blood test since my white count was alarmingly low. Additionally, he advised me to reevaluate my job. He was convinced that the vertigo, hives, and low blood count were all manifestations of my body's response to the stress and grief I was experiencing.

He believed I could manage this without medication. He said that stress and anxiety are natural parts of life and that learning to navigate the ups and downs is a necessary skill. Not only can coping skills prevent a lifetime of reliance on medication, but they are also effective in so many other areas of life. The realization that I had the power to change my life felt great, but I did not know where to begin. It meant embarking on a journey of introspection and facing the realities of what wasn't working and what needed changing, which felt overwhelming. He suggested that I start by trying meditation.

Determined to equip myself with the tools to manage this, I immersed myself in yoga and meditation. I attended classes on herbs, natural medicine, spirituality, nutrition, and researched the mind-body connection. This path led me to study energy healing, Reiki, reflexology, aromatherapy, and, best of all, Ayurveda. In working with an Ayurvedic doctor who later became my mentor, I was able to not only manage the anxiety but also put it into perspective.

Another critical step was facing the bigger issue, my job. I had a meeting with Human Resources and then met with my manager. To my surprise, the conversation went smoothly. We both agreed that we were not the right fit for each other. This experience taught me a valuable lesson: confront your fears, they may not be as bad as they seem!

I transitioned to another department and spent many years working there with wonderful people. A few months later, my mother passed away, and the last time I experienced those hives was on the day we laid her to rest. Once my work situation changed, the bouts of vertigo and shortness of breath ceased. This set me on a path that grew into a deep passion, one I now share with others to support their own healing journeys.

Keep in mind that anxiety is a universal part of being human, something that affects all of us at some point in our lives. The pivotal question becomes; how do we effectively navigate it? Recent years have witnessed a significant spotlight on mental health, with many people in the public eye bravely sharing their struggles. Statistics show that 43% of adults reported increased anxiety in 2024, up from 37% in 2023. Younger adults, particularly those between 18 and 34, have identified social connection as a significant factor influencing their mental health. These trends underscore the urgent need for comprehensive mental health care that supports each person physically, mentally, and emotionally.

We must eliminate the stigma around mental health and treat it the same as any other medical condition, like diabetes or heart disease. While treatment options have come a long way, integrating traditional medicine with holistic approaches can offer powerful and lasting support.

This book is my invitation to you, a clear, compassionate roadmap grounded in my years of personal and professional experience. In this revised edition, I've integrated the latest research and healing strategies to reflect the evolving understanding of anxiety. My goal is to provide practical, accessible tools to support your growth, healing, and resilience.

Even though this book is called The Holistic Root to Managing Anxiety, I want to emphasize that I completely respect anyone's decision to use medication and do not judge that choice. Finding a trusted doctor who listens and supports you is a crucial step in your healing journey. Many clients start with medication and later adopt a more integrative approach. The good news is that an increasing number of alternative options are now available for long-term anxiety management. Ultimately, healing comes from addressing the root causes of your anxiety and discovering the approach that feels right for you.

As an Integrative Nutritionist, Board-Certified Health & Wellness Coach, Functional Nutrition Coach, Certified Ayurveda Practitioner, Herbalist, and Registered Yoga & Meditation Teacher, my passion is combining time-tested traditions with modern science to empower you to reclaim your health.

How to Use This Book

This book is designed to be practical and approachable. Whether you're dealing with anxiety or want to strengthen your ability to handle life's stressors, start small. Try the DIY remedies at your own pace. The goal isn't perfection, but progress, small, consistent steps that shift how you relate to stress and anxiety.

Engage actively with the tools provided. Notice how your body and mind respond. The book offers a variety of strategies, from nutrition and therapy to yoga and mindfulness, so you can find what truly works for you.

What This Book Can Do for You

This book is for anyone who feels the weight of anxiety, whether from everyday stress or deeper-rooted issues. It's for those looking for a way out of the constant cycle of fear and unease. It's for those ready to take charge of their health and well-being and are open to the healing potential of an integrated approach. Whether you are new to these practices or have been on a wellness path for years, the tools in this book will support you.

It is important to remember that there is no one-size-fits-all solution to anxiety. It's a deeply personal experience, and what works for one person may not work for another. Healing is a gradual process that requires time, patience, and self-compassion. With the right tools and guidance, you can begin to shift the course of your life toward lasting health and well-being.

The solution lies within each individual and how they navigate life's challenges. Even if you do not currently struggle with anxiety, understanding how to manage life stressors helps create a happier, healthier life. Our bodies possess incredible restorative potential, and with proper guidance, healing is always within our reach. Always remember, the power lies within you!

With gratitude and healing,

Maria

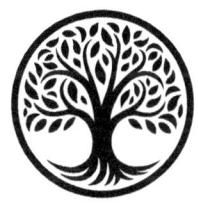

"Be the change you want to see in the world."
— Mahatma Gandhi

CHAPTER 1

What is Anxiety?

Anxiety is something we all experience from time to time. It might show up as a tightness in the chest before a difficult conversation, stress when checking the news, or restlessness late at night when your thoughts won't slow down. Whether it's worrying about your kids, health, finances, or just getting through the day, anxiety can arise when life feels uncertain. But when anxiety becomes chronic or disproportionate, it disrupts daily life, making you feel like something is always about to go wrong, even when everything seems fine. While some handle it more easily than others, acknowledging anxiety is the first step, and from there, it's a process of uncovering its underlying causes. Ignoring these feelings over time can harm your health and lead to more serious conditions.

There are several types of anxiety disorders, including Generalized Anxiety Disorder (GAD), social anxiety disorder, panic disorder, and specific phobias. GAD, for instance, is marked by persistent and often irrational worry that lasts for six months or more.

Symptoms can vary widely, including excessive worry, restlessness, irritability, difficulty concentrating, muscle tension, digestive disturbances, dizziness, fatigue, and sleep disruption. While some people trace their anxiety to specific stressors, others find it harder to pinpoint a source. In today's fast-paced world, with everything constantly changing and the never-ending stream of information from our phones and news feeds, it can feel like the weight of the world is always on our shoulders. Women are nearly twice as likely as men to suffer from anxiety, and an estimated forty million adults in the U.S. are affected each year.

Traditionally, anxiety is treated with a mix of medication and therapy. While medications can help many people, they often come with side effects. These treatments generally focus on managing symptoms rather than addressing the underlying causes. As someone who supports an integrative approach, I believe it's crucial to explore the root causes of anxiety. Many ancient wisdom traditions have understood the deep connection between the mind and body for thousands of years.

Dr. Gabor Maté, a Canadian physician specializing in family medicine, palliative care, and addiction treatment, has spent over twenty years working with patients facing complex challenges, including trauma, mental illness, and substance use. He is the best-selling author of books such as "When the Body Says No" and "The Myth of Normal", which explore the deep connections between emotional stress, early life experiences, and physical health. Dr. Maté approaches anxiety not as a standalone mental illness, but as a symptom of deeper emotional wounds, often originating in early childhood. He believes many people develop anxiety when, as children, they feel unsafe expressing their authentic emotions or needs. To maintain the connection with caregivers, they unconsciously learn to suppress parts of themselves, becoming hyper-vigilant, overly responsible, or emotionally disconnected in the process. While this survival adaptation may be protective in childhood, it later becomes a source of chronic tension and anxiety.

Dr. Maté's therapeutic method, known as Compassionate Inquiry, focuses on gently uncovering the stories and beliefs we've internalized, especially the ones operating beneath the surface. The goal isn't to "get rid" of anxiety, but to understand what it's trying to say.

Instead of only treating symptoms, Dr. Maté emphasizes healing through connection: reconnecting with the body's sensations, with emotions we've long buried, and with safe, supportive relationships. He encourages people to become curious about their anxiety, asking not "What's wrong with me?" but "What happened to me?" Through this lens, anxiety becomes not a flaw, but a clue pointing us back to places within ourselves that need compassion, safety, and healing.

In his book Anxiety Rx, Dr. Russell Kennedy, a physician and neuroscientist who has personally struggled with anxiety, introduces the idea that anxiety is often a mental reaction to something deeper, which he calls "alarm." This alarm isn't just a feeling. Its unresolved emotional pain stored in the body, often dating back to childhood trauma. According to Dr. Kennedy, the mind senses this discomfort and interprets it as anxiety, trying to make sense of it with worry, rumination, or fear-based narratives. However, until the underlying "alarm" is addressed, those mental patterns will persist, regardless of how much cognitive therapy we pursue.

One of the key players in Dr. Kennedy's model is the vagus nerve, a long, wandering nerve that connects the brain to the heart, lungs, and digestive tract. It's central to the parasympathetic nervous system, which governs our ability to rest, digest, and feel safe. When this nerve is dysregulated, often due to chronic stress or unresolved trauma, we may find ourselves stuck in states of hypervigilance, shutdown, or dissociation. This dysregulation can manifest as physical symptoms we commonly associate with anxiety: a racing heart, shallow breath, nausea, or a "gut feeling" of dread.

Dr. Kennedy emphasizes the importance of practices that reconnect with the body to resolve the alarm at its source. These may include slow, diaphragmatic breathing to stimulate the vagus nerve, mindful movement, self-compassion meditations, or simply placing a hand on the chest or belly to signal safety. By engaging the body and soothing the nervous system, we can begin to unwind the loop of mind-based anxiety and return to a grounded state of calm.

Anxiety disorders are highly treatable, yet only a fraction of those affected seek treatment. Left unmanaged, anxiety can evolve into depression and compromise the immune system. This underscores the importance of acquiring skills to minimize stress and recognizing anxiety early, along with implementing coping strategies.

New York City psychologist Dr. Debbie Rothschild emphasizes that anxiety is a combination of nature and nurture, shaped by both genetic predisposition and environmental factors. She notes that anxiety often mirrors patterns seen in parents, highlighting the significant impact of our upbringing. However, it's essential to recognize that we can alter these patterns. While genetics may play a role, adopting a mindset that change is impossible can lead to helplessness. Epigenetics teaches us that lifestyle choices and mindset can influence the expression of our genes.

Dr. Rothschild also points out that a moderate level of anxiety can motivate us, helping us focus and grow. In my own experience, anxiety pushed me toward positive change, though when it escalates into a disorder, it can make daily functioning difficult. Early recognition and proactive steps are key to healing.

Acupuncturist Phyllis Shapiro reminds us that life's stressors are inevitable, but how we respond is within our control. She stresses that many effective approaches to anxiety don't rely on pharmaceuticals, and that achieving long-term success requires gradual adjustments to our lives. Anxiety must be addressed in the present moment, allowing yourself to experience it without suppression. While quick fixes, such as medication, might offer temporary relief, they often don't address the root causes. Whether through therapy, medication, or other methods, the key is finding what works for you and committing to consistent compassionate healing.

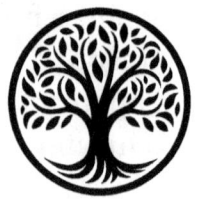

> "We have more technology but less time for ourselves."
>
> — JON KABAT-ZINN

CHAPTER 2

Social Media and the Pace of Modern Life

Those close to me are well aware of my aversion to social media. While it can facilitate connections with distant family and friends, especially during the COVID-19 pandemic, it's a double-edged sword. It served as a lifeline during the pandemic but also became a breeding ground for conspiracy theories, misinformation, online harassment, and vitriol.

The influence of social media on our interactions, information consumption, and daily lives is undeniable. Depending on its use, the impact can be positive or negative. Despite the opportunities and advantages, mounting evidence suggests that it is a factor in the rise of anxiety.

Social media often offers a skewed perspective of reality, with people sharing only what appears to be the happiest moments of their lives. There has been considerable research on the psychological effects of the infamous "like" button.

It can foster a culture of self-promotion and superficiality. It encourages users to present a carefully curated, idealized version of themselves to seek approval from others. This can make people feel like they're not being themselves and create pressure to fit in with societal expectations. Research also shows that it often leads to self-comparison and negative emotions, and let's be honest, it doesn't always reflect reality either.

Studies reveal that college students who spent more time on social media reported increased levels of anxiety and depression, along with more frequent bouts of FOMO (Fear of Missing Out). FOMO is something many people feel, especially with social media constantly showing us what everyone else is doing. This can lead to heightened levels of anxiety and stress, as users feel compelled to incessantly check their feeds to stay abreast of the latest news and events. It perpetuates social comparison and instills a constant need for acceptance from others.

The like button can potentially foster addictive behaviors by triggering the brain's reward system, akin to the effects of drugs and other addictive substances.

False information spreads rapidly on social media platforms when accompanied by numerous likes. Researchers suggest it creates an effect wherein users are more inclined to believe and share information that has already received validation from others.

During the COVID-19 pandemic, social media played a crucial role in preventing many from descending into the depths of loneliness and depression. While it can never replace the warmth of face-to-face communication and a comforting hug, it provided solace in knowing that we were all in this together and could share our stories.

One of the major concerns is its potential to exacerbate feelings of social isolation and loneliness. Vivek Murthy, the former U.S. Surgeon General, has publicly addressed the impact of social media on mental health, including its role in contributing to anxiety. Murthy discusses how social media can intensify sensations of isolation and loneliness, stating that "the more time we spend on social media, the more likely we are to be depressed and anxious."

Another study conducted by researchers at the University of Pennsylvania found that limiting social media use to thirty minutes per day led to a notable reduction in feelings of anxiety and depression. The study involved 143 undergraduate students who initially reported high levels of both. Participants were randomly assigned to either restrict their social media time or continue using it as usual. After three weeks, those who limited their use reported significantly lower levels of anxiety and depression compared to the control group.

Limiting time spent on devices can indeed reduce anxiety. However, the prevailing work culture in America, which demands constant connectivity, poses a significant challenge. The boundary between work and personal time has become increasingly blurred, with pressure to be available around the clock, often driven by the fear of losing one's job. This has led to a collective addiction to perpetual productivity, causing us to lose touch with the ability to simply be.

Many find themselves constantly in motion, fearing the discomfort that arises when they pause and confront their thoughts and emotions. The constant busyness serves as a distraction from deeper introspection.

As a society, we've struggled to manage our lives and the accompanying stressors. It's not necessarily the stress itself but rather how we cope with it that determines its impact on our well-being. Neglecting to acknowledge and address anxiety can potentially lead to more significant challenges in the future.

Even more concerning is the growing link between increased social media and technology use and the rise in depressive symptoms and suicide rates among adolescents in the U.S. A 2018 study (Twenge et al., 2018) found that excessive screen time was strongly associated with these troubling trends. For many young people, the constant pressure to stay connected, keep up, and present an idealized version of themselves online can take a serious toll on their mental and emotional well-being.

Striking a balance is key. The initial step is to cultivate mindfulness regarding the amount of time devoted to social media. What's the worst that could happen if you took a break and limited screen time? Begin gradually, perhaps by going for a short walk without your phone and increase the time each day. Set an alarm a few hours before bedtime to power down your devices and keep them out of your bedroom. Change unfolds gradually, and over time, you'll be surprised at how much more enriching and fulfilling your life can become. You may even discover other hobbies and things that bring you joy.

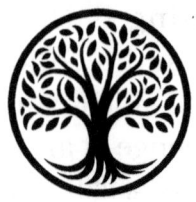

> "The gateways to wisdom and knowledge are always open."
>
> — Louise Hay

CHAPTER 3

Acupuncture

Acupuncture, an ancient Chinese medical practice dating back over 3,000 years, aims to unblock the vital life energy known as chi or qi (pronounced "chee"). The human body has over 2,000 acupuncture points situated along fourteen major meridians. These meridians serve as pathways that connect acupuncture points, facilitating the flow of energy throughout the body. When this energy flow encounters blockages or disruptions, it can lead to illness. Therefore, restoring the natural flow of life energy is essential in restoring the body's balance. The process involves gently inserting needles at specific meridian points on the body, which, I assure you, is not painful at all. In fact, it's quite relaxing.

Chinese medicine integrates mind, body, and spirit in diagnosis. During my struggle with anxiety, acupuncture was very helpful. As a result, I've recommended it to numerous clients dealing with both anxiety and depression.

Phyllis Shapiro, a Licensed Acupuncturist and Traditional Chinese Medicine Doctor based in New York City, emphasizes that:

"According to Traditional Chinese Medicine (TCM), anxiety is considered an underlying factor in many health conditions. It particularly affects the liver meridian system, which plays a key role in ensuring the smooth and balanced flow of chi, or life-force energy. When this flow becomes disrupted, it can lead to imbalances throughout the body, as the circulation of energy and fluids supports detoxification and overall healing."

Regardless of the specific symptoms or condition, calming the spirit and creating regular moments of stillness, especially in alignment with the body's natural sleep cycle, is essential to the healing process. During restful sleep, the body carries out repair and renewal functions. When anxiety interferes with that rest, the body's ability to recover is significantly diminished. To support this process, calming herbal remedies can be used to encourage relaxation, reduce tension, and promote more restorative sleep.

Dr. Shapiro's diagnostic process involves a thorough inquiry. She pays close attention to how patients communicate, noting their speech patterns, tone, and appearance, as well as observing their movements and reactions. This meticulous approach aims to uncover the root cause of their anxiety. What a patient shares is particularly significant. Unlike conventional medical practitioners, Chinese medicine practitioners invest more time in listening to their patients and seeking to identify the underlying issues that require attention. Dr. Andrew Weil stated that, given enough time, a patient may be able to effectively self-diagnose, emphasizing the value of deep listening in the diagnostic process.

What distinguishes Chinese Medicine, and what I find to be a logical approach to healing, is the open-mindedness in pinpointing the root cause of an ailment. This consideration ultimately contributes to a more comprehensive and accurate diagnosis.

It's worth noting that many acupuncturists may be covered by insurance, so it's advisable to check with your insurance company to determine if you have coverage.

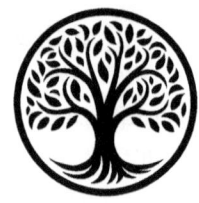

> "Smell is a potent wizard that transports you across thousands of miles and all the years you have lived."
>
> — Helen Keller

CHAPTER 4

Aromatherapy

Aromatherapy is a healing treatment utilizing the therapeutic properties of essential oils to nurture the mind, body, spirit, and surroundings. This ancient tradition boasts a rich history spanning millennia across diverse cultures, including Arabia, China, India, Egypt, Greece, Israel, Tibet, and eventually Europe, where it proved effective in various uses, spanning from perfumery to the embalming process. Every corner of the world has integrated aromatherapy into its practices, whether for medicinal purposes, rituals, or the creation of beautiful fragrances.

Essential oils offer benefits for both physical and emotional well-being that go beyond their pleasant scents. They are made through steam distillation from flowers, roots, seeds, berries, bark, leaves, resin, needles, and fruit peels. They are insoluble in water and highly concentrated.

They can help with a wide range of issues, including stress reduction, enhanced immune function, increased vitality, pain relief, improved memory, and digestive support. They can also help stabilize mood, enhance meditation, and contain compounds that can fight viral and bacterial infections. Many cosmetic companies are incorporating essential oils into their skincare products due to their beneficial effects on skin conditions and non-toxic approach to skincare.

The way inhaling or applying essential oils affects our health occurs through the olfactory system, which is directly connected to the hypothalamus, a part of the brain that links to the limbic system, which governs emotions, behavior, and memory. The minute you inhale an essential oil that you love, your nervous system begins to respond, your breath deepens, your shoulders drop, and your mind starts to shift into a more relaxed, grounded state.

Ancient civilizations such as the Egyptians, Greeks, and later Europeans discovered that marjoram and cypress helped alleviate grief and sadness by strengthening the brain and supporting the ability to move forward in life.

How do you feel when you smell fresh baking or home-cooked meals? These scents can transport you to happy or sad memories, depending on whether the memory is positive or negative. Either way, they evoke an emotional response.

Given that it takes a large quantity of plant material to produce a small amount of essential oil, always use the oils responsibly. Less is more when it comes to using essential oils. For example, it takes petals from forty to fifty roses to produce a single drop of rose oil.

Carrier Oil

A carrier oil, also called a base oil, is mixed with essential oils before applying to the skin. Because essential oils are highly concentrated, diluting them with a carrier oil ensures safe and gentle use. My preferred carrier oils are sesame and almond, both valued for their antioxidant properties and excellent absorption. However, many other options work well, including coconut, sunflower, apricot, avocado, jojoba, rosehip seed, castor, grapeseed, hazelnut, and olive oil.

Always choose 100% pure essential oils. While some essential oils can be applied undiluted, I recommend diluting all essential oils with a carrier oil to minimize irritation and enhance safety.

For blending, use a one-ounce amber or blue glass bottle. These colors protect the oils from sunlight, which can degrade their quality. Stored properly in colored glass, an oil blend can last up to a year. Avoid plastic containers, as they can react with the oils and compromise their effectiveness.

Start by adding fifteen drops of essential oil into the bottle. These drops can include up to five different essential oils blended together. Next, fill the rest of the bottle with a carrier oil. Sesame oil is a great choice for managing anxiety due to its grounding properties. Secure the cap tightly and gently roll the bottle between your palms to thoroughly mix the oils.

Essential oils and bottles are widely available at health food stores or online. Additional resources can be found at the end of this book.

Mixing your own essential oil blends is also a fun way to tap into your creativity. You can customize a blend to suit your current needs and take it with you for massage or reflexology sessions. I enjoy making my own blends because it allows me to tailor them specifically to how I'm feeling in the moment.

I love using an aromatherapy diffuser, which is a device that releases essential oils into the air as a fine mist or vapor. It works by combining water and essential oils, then dispersing the blend through ultrasonic vibrations, heat, or a fan. This process fills the space with the aromatic and therapeutic benefits of the oils.

Diffusing essential oils in the evening can promote relaxation, while using them in a workspace can help boost energy and improve focus. Chamomile and lavender are popular choices for diffusing in a child's room to soothe colic, provided there are no allergies. When adding essential oils to a diffuser, they should be used undiluted.

Types of Diffusers

- **Ultrasonic diffusers** use water and ultrasonic vibrations to break down essential oils into small particles, dispersing them as a fine mist into the air. This is the most common type of diffuser and is both inexpensive and practical.
- **Nebulizing diffusers** use pressurized air or gas to break down the oils into tiny particles, creating a more concentrated aroma without the need for water or heat.
- **Heat diffusers** rely on heat, typically from a candle or electricity, to evaporate essential oils into the air. However, heat may alter the chemical composition of the oils.
- **Evaporative diffusers** involve a fan blowing air through a pad or filter containing essential oils, causing the oils to evaporate more quickly. These can be used in the car.

Lastly, don't underestimate the power of a bath! While our fast-paced lives don't always allow for it, taking a bath when stressed offers a much-needed escape. Add five to six drops of essential oil to the bathwater after filling the tub and indulge in a twenty-minute soak.

Here are some of my favorite essential oils for easing anxiety. I've included a mix so there's something for everyone, regardless of the scents you're drawn to. Keep in mind to always dilute them with a carrier oil before applying to your skin. And don't be afraid to experiment. Mix a few and create a calming blend that's uniquely you!

Lavender (Lavandula angustifolia)

Lavender is an incredibly versatile oil that should be in every household. Its historical use in taming lions and tigers attests to its remarkable calming properties. Lavender is renowned for its ability to soothe anxiety, insomnia, depression, bolster the immune system, and aid in healing skin lesions. When you're feeling anxious, stressed, or nervous, place a few drops in your hand with a teaspoon of almond or sesame oil, rub them together, and take a few deep breaths. Alternatively, apply a few drops of the blend to the inside of your wrists, which will be absorbed into your body. Lavender is a great, all-natural alternative to chemically laden perfumes.

Another great tip is to apply lavender (diluted with a carrier oil) to the soles of your feet before bedtime to encourage deep, restful sleep. Studies show it can increase time spent in deep sleep. I also love adding lavender oil to my bath for relaxation.

For a simple sleep aid, mix 10 drops of lavender oil with 4 ounces of water in a spray bottle and mist your pillows before bed. It's also a good idea to keep a bottle in your car, and if you feel a bout of road rage coming on, take a whiff!

Roman Chamomile (Chamaemelum nobile)

First documented in the mid-16th century, Roman chamomile is a small perennial herb cherished by the Egyptians, Greeks, and Romans. It makes for a delightful addition to any garden. There are two primary types: Roman and German chamomile. For its calming properties, Roman chamomile is the preferred choice. This herb offers support to the nervous and digestive systems. It also serves as a remedy for headaches and migraines. Apply a few drops, mixed with a carrier oil, to your temples. It is also an excellent choice for a soothing massage blend or use in the bath, providing a deeply relaxing experience. Diffusing chamomile in a child's room can relieve colic and promote a sense of calm.

Rose (Rosa damascena)

Who can resist the beautiful scent of a lovely rose? Rose oil is renowned for fostering harmony and well-being, soothing frayed nerves, and may help relieve depression. You can use it in the same manner as the other oils. While it may be a bit pricier because it takes forty to fifty roses to yield a single drop of rose essential oil, its benefits are worth every penny! Consider purchasing oil that is already diluted in a carrier oil for a more budget-friendly option. This way, you can enjoy the benefits without breaking the bank.

Neroli (Citrus aurantium)

One of my favorites is this exquisite oil derived from the bitter orange tree. It owes its name to the Italian Princess Nerola, who introduced it to Italy for her personal use as a perfume. Like rose, the extraction process contributes to its higher price tag. Neroli is renowned for its calming effects on anxiety, its ability to facilitate restful sleep, and its potential to alleviate symptoms of depression and PMS. For a truly tranquil experience, add a few drops of neroli oil to your bath and let the stress melt away. Additionally, inhaling a single drop of neroli, blended with carrier oil, can relieve headaches.

Lemon Balm (Melissa officinalis)

Lemon Balm, also known as Melissa, is one of those gentle, calming herbs that can significantly aid in improving sleep and mood. It's great for winding down and may even help lift feelings of sadness. Try mixing it with sesame oil and gently massaging it onto your abdomen to help ease menstrual cramps. Just make sure your bottle is pure lemon balm, not lemon oil (they're different!). You can also diffuse it in a child's room to help them relax and sleep more peacefully.

Jatamansi (Nardostachys jatamansi)

Jatamansi oil, also recognized as Himalayan spikenard, holds a special place in Ayurvedic tradition across India. This oil has a remarkably calming and grounding effect, helping you feel more balanced, supporting better sleep, and providing true comfort during challenging emotional times. Try diluting it with a carrier oil and applying it to the soles of your feet or the crown of your head before bed. It's a simple way to invite in deeper sleep and more peaceful dreams.

Vetiver (Vetiveria zizanioides)

Vetiver carries the essence of the earth. Its grounding and calming properties make it a popular choice for perfume. It provides a soothing embrace for the mind and body, facilitating deep, restorative sleep. Additionally, it can aid in concentration and is a delightful addition to a carrier oil for massage or undiluted in a diffuser in the evening to promote sleep.

Ylang Ylang Complete (Cananga odorata var. genuina)

Ylang Ylang is a beautiful floral essence renowned for its ability to soothe anger, alleviate anxiety, and foster emotional equilibrium. It has also been known to lower blood pressure. Ylang Ylang boasts healing properties for the skin and is often included in skincare blends. When combined with other oils, especially those known for their supportive effects on depression, such as neroli, rose, bergamot, geranium, lavender, jasmine, and sweet orange, it creates a lovely blend with enhanced benefits. I mix it with almond oil and use it as perfume.

Frankincense (Boswellia serrata)

Frankincense is one of the most widely used essential oils, valued for its numerous benefits in traditional cultures that span thousands of years. Revered for its potent ability to uplift and bring clarity to the body and mind, frankincense oil has been used for thousands of years for prayer and meditation. It fosters a positive and serene atmosphere within your living space, transforming your home into a tranquil sanctuary.

> **CAUTION:** Avoid applying essential oils to infants, even if diluted. While essential oils can benefit colicky children in a diffuser, seeking guidance from a certified aromatherapist before use is crucial. If you are pregnant, the safest method for using essential oils is through a diffuser.
>
> Remember that certain essential oils, such as citrus oils, are phototoxic, meaning they can cause reactions when exposed to sunlight or other forms of light. It's advised to avoid sun exposure after using citrus oils.

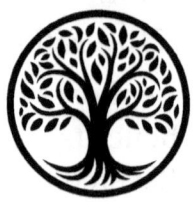

> "A physician who fails to enter the body of a patient with the lamp of Knowledge and understanding can never treat diseases. He should first study all factors, including the environment, which influence a patient's disease, and then prescribe treatment. It is more important to prevent the occurrence of disease than to seek cure."
>
> — CHARAKA SAMHITA

CHAPTER 5

Ayurveda

Ayurveda is an ancient system of medicine originating from India, with a history spanning over 5,000 years. It is the sister science to yoga. Ayur means "life," and Veda means "science" or "knowledge," translating to "the science or knowledge of life." Unlike the standard definition of health, which is "the state of being free from illness or injury," Ayurvedic philosophy believes that a harmonious balance between the body, mind, spirit, and environment characterizes optimal health. Thus, the primary goal of Ayurveda is to maintain harmony among all these elements.

When that harmony is disrupted, it can lead to illness and disease. It's a system of medicine that recognizes each person as an individual, understanding that two people with the same ailment may need different treatments based on their unique constitution.

Traditionally, there has been a separation between medical care for the body and spiritual practices for the soul. However, we now understand that the mind, body, and spirit are intricately interconnected and function as a unified whole. It is impossible to isolate emotions from illness or illness from emotions. For instance, being in love can lead to "butterflies in your stomach." At the same time, stress can manifest as physical symptoms, such as stomach discomfort or headaches, illustrating the direct connection between our emotional and physical health.

Western medicine is undoubtedly amazing. If you're having a heart attack or break a bone, you're not calling your herbalist! However, it often takes a narrow view, focusing on the illness rather than the person as a whole. It tends to focus on symptoms and leans toward a one-size-fits-all approach. Ayurveda, on the other hand, looks at the bigger picture. What works for one person might not work for another. Typically, a conventional doctor examines the issue and prescribes medication or recommends a procedure. While this approach is sometimes necessary, going deeper to uncover the root cause of the problem encourages patients to connect their physical imbalance with their broader life circumstances. It forces us to go inward and reflect. Ancient traditions have maintained that our cells hold wisdom and memories, emphasizing that the issue may resurface unless the root cause is addressed. Lifestyle, career, diet, and relationships can all contribute to illness, necessitating deeper introspection for understanding and resolution.

Ayurveda believes that the origin of illness lies in the mind, which subsequently manifests in the body. It believes that our thoughts are the root of our anxiety and depression.

Ruminating on negative or destructive thoughts can make them our reality. But when we treat ourselves with love and compassion and focus on positive thoughts, those become our truth instead. Ayurveda examines our connection with nature and our soul, two aspects of our existence that modern life often overlooks.

So, How Does Ayurveda Facilitate Healing?

Ayurveda helps you achieve and maintain vibrant health by identifying your unique dosha, or constitution, which serves as your personalized blueprint for a healthy life. *Doshas* are the fundamental bio-energies or life forces that govern the physical and mental processes of the body. There are three primary doshas, comprised of the five elements, known as:

- **Vata** (air and ether)
- **Pitta** (fire and water)
- **Kapha** (earth and water)

Understanding your *dosha* provides insight into your innate nature, shedding light on why certain foods may not align with you, why you prefer one season over another, and which ailments you are predisposed to. It serves as a guide to an appropriate diet, exercise routines, and lifestyle practices for your specific body type.

While everyone embodies a combination of all three *doshas*, most people have one predominant *dosha*, often coupled with a secondary one. We can achieve balance in our *doshas* through proper diet, daily routines, meditation, harmonizing with nature, attuning to our senses and the seasons, herbal remedies, body treatments, and aromatherapy.

In Ayurveda, anxiety is attributed to an imbalance in the Vata *dosha*, which comprises the elements of air and ether. Vata is known for its light, dry, and constantly moving nature. When balanced, Vata brings quick thinking, creativity, inspiration, and high energy. However, when it's out of balance, it can leave you feeling scattered, anxious, unfocused, and ungrounded, like life is moving a little too fast. Its dry quality can show up as dry skin, constipation, or exhaustion, while its lightness and constant movement often lead to restlessness, racing thoughts, and difficulty sleeping. This imbalance is also associated with conditions such as ADHD, which is considered Vata-related. Elevated Vata can lead to an overactive nervous system, potentially causing insomnia. When I work with clients experiencing anxiety or teach meditation in classes, I often hear, "I can't meditate because my mind is always racing." That is the classic Vata personality.

The way to balance Vata is through a calm and grounding approach. This involves establishing a consistent daily routine, including regular mealtimes, waking and going to sleep at the same time, and maintaining a steady work routine. For a better night's sleep, it helps to keep your phone and TV out of the bedroom and aim to turn off the lights by 10 p.m. I know it's tough, given how connected we all are, but taking the time to unwind makes a difference. Meditating and expressing gratitude before bedtime can further enhance a transition into a relaxed sleep state. Make sure you are comfortably warm, even in warmer weather. Diffusing essential oils in the room can contribute to a peaceful night's sleep. Additionally, refraining from eating after 5 p.m. allows the body ample time for digestion. Eating late disrupts the body's digestive process, preventing it from adequately preparing to eliminate toxins and manage stress, which can disturb a good night's sleep.

Ayurveda also recommends body treatments called Shirodhara and Abhyanga, which are highly beneficial for anxiety and overall health and well-being.

Shirodhara is an Ayurvedic treatment derived from the Sanskrit words *"shiro" (meaning head)* and *"dhara" (meaning flow)*. It involves the gentle, continuous pouring of warm herbal oil over the forehead for thirty to sixty minutes, targeting the area known as the "third eye" or *Ajna Chakra*, which is believed to be the seat of human consciousness. This practice can:

Calms the Nervous System: The steady stream of warm oil stimulates the third eye and forehead, helping to calm the hypothalamus and regulate the pituitary gland's activity, which in turn helps to relax the nervous system.

Reduces Stress Hormones: The rhythmic flow of oil can lower cortisol levels, the primary stress hormone, which is often elevated in individuals experiencing chronic stress and anxiety.

Promotes Deep Relaxation: It induces deep relaxation, similar to meditation, which helps reduce anxiety and promotes mental clarity.

Improves Sleep Quality: *Shirodhara* is known to enhance sleep quality by helping with insomnia and promoting deeper, more restful sleep.

Balances Doshas: *Shirodhara* helps balance the doshas (body energies), particularly **Vata** and **Pitta**, which, when imbalanced, can contribute to anxiety and stress.

Enhances Mood: The treatment can increase levels of serotonin and dopamine in the brain, neurotransmitters associated with mood regulation and overall well-being.

Reduces Headaches and Tension: *Shirodhara* can reduce headaches and tension, often associated with anxiety, by relaxing the muscles and nerves around the head and neck.

Detoxifies the Mind and Body: The herbal oils used are often infused with detoxifying ingredients, helping to clear toxins that may contribute to anxiety.

Abhyanga

Abhyanga is a full-body massage using warm herbal oils. The word *Abhyanga* means "massaging the body's limbs" in Sanskrit. This treatment rejuvenates and detoxifies the body while promoting a sense of grounding and connection with the earth. You can perform the treatment on yourself or visit a massage therapist.

Abhyanga is an integral part of the Ayurvedic daily routine. The oils are not just spread over the skin but are deeply massaged into the tissues, targeting key *marma* or pressure points, similar to acupuncture. It enhances blood circulation throughout the body while providing a calming effect that deepens the connection between the mind, body, and spirit. It releases what Ayurveda refers to as *ama* (deep toxins), improves skin texture and tone, moisturizes the skin, reduces muscle stiffness and joint pain, strengthens the immune system, reduces stress, and promotes mental tranquility.

Nourishing your body with herbal oils ensures that both your body and soul feel loved and that your chakras remain in balance. The oils are chosen based on the individual's *dosha* and health condition.

An Ayurveda practitioner can guide you toward physical, emotional, and spiritual well-being. This heightened self-awareness empowers you to take control of your health.

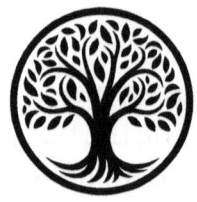

> "Health depends on being in harmony with our souls."
>
> — Dr. Edward Bach

CHAPTER 6

Bach Flower Essences

A homeopath and bacteriologist named Dr. Edward Bach developed the Bach Original Flower Remedies in the 1920s as a holistic approach to healing the mind and emotions. Dr. Bach grew disillusioned with the medical establishment's focus on treating disease rather than the whole person. He believed that emotional distress, like anxiety, stemmed from imbalances in the body's energy. To address this, he identified thirty-eight specific emotional states and created a corresponding set of thirty-eight flower remedies, each designed to help restore emotional harmony and inner balance.

Several studies suggest that Bach Flower Essences can help ease anxiety, stress, and depression while supporting emotional clarity and resilience. They're considered safe, with no known side effects, making them a gentle and natural choice for anyone seeking emotional relief.

Made from non-toxic flowering plants and trees, these essences are safe for everyone, including infants, seniors, and even pets. Unlike pharmaceuticals or herbs, they don't interact chemically with other treatments and aren't addictive.

A 2016 study by the University of Miami School of Nursing and Health Studies found that people who used Bach Flower Essences experienced a significant reduction in symptoms of anxiety and depression compared to those who did not. The study involved a sample of fifty participants over six weeks. Those using the essences reported notable improvements in anxiety, stress, and depression, suggesting that Bach Flower Remedies may be a helpful natural alternative for those seeking emotional relief.

Another study published in the *Journal of Complementary and Alternative Medicine* in 2011 found that using Bach Flower Essences was associated with reduced anxiety and stress levels in eighty people. The study lasted for eight weeks, and participants reported a significant improvement in their overall emotional state and reduced anxiety symptoms.

Below are the thirty-eight negative states, along with the corresponding Bach remedy that supports each one. If you experience more than one of these emotions, you can mix the remedies to make a personal formula, or you can go to the Bach website listed at the end of this book, which has a "remedy chooser" to help you find the remedy you need. Millions of people use Bach remedies successfully in sixty-six countries worldwide.

Bach also makes a blend called **Rescue Remedy**. It is a blend of five of the thirty-eight remedies: Rock Rose for terror and panic, Impatiens for irritation and impatience, Clematis for inattentiveness, Star of Bethlehem for shock, and Cherry Plum for irrational thoughts. Keep a bottle of it handy in your bag or pocket for those moments of stress. Rescue Remedy can also be used on animals. Given its safety and effectiveness, this is an excellent initial approach for those unfamiliar with complementary or holistic therapies.

Thirty-Eight Emotional States and Corresponding Bach Remedy	
Emotional State	**Bach Remedy**
Emotional State of Terror	Rock Rose
Fear of the Unknown	Mimulus
Fear of Mental Incapability	Cherry Plum
Fear and Worry of the Unknown	Aspen
Concern and Fear for Others	Red Chestnut
Feeling Aloof or Proud	Water Violet
Being Impatient	Impatiens
Self-Absorption	Heather
Dreamy and Disconnection from Present	Clematis
Living in the Past	Honeysuckle
Apathy and Resignation	Wild Rose
Lack of Vitality and Energy	Olive
Mental Incongruency	White Chestnut
Gloom and Doom	Mustard
Repeating Past Mistakes	Chestnut Bud
Lacking Confidence	Larch
Feelings of Guilt	Pine
Overwhelmed by Responsibility	Elm
Mental Anguish	Sweet Chestnut

Thirty-Eight Emotional States and Corresponding Bach Remedy

Emotional State	Bach Remedy
Shock Recovery	Star of Bethlehem
Resentment	Willow
Energy to Continue When Feeling Exhaustion	Oak
Self-Hatred and Lack of Cleanliness	Crab Apple
Need for External Validation	Cerato
Indecisiveness	Scleranthus
Despondent With Feelings of Discouragement	Gentian
Feelings of Despair and Hopelessness	Gorse
Energy for Beginnings	Hornbeam
Life Path Uncertainty	Wild Oat
Acting Brave When Mentally Tormented	Agrimony
Subservience and Lack of Will	Centaury
Wanting Protection from Change and External Influences	Walnut
Feelings of Hate, Jealousy, and Envy	Holly
Possessiveness	Chicory
Over-Enthusiastic	Vervain
Inflexible with Domineering Tendencies	Vine
Intolerant Attitude	Beech
Self-Denial and Repressiveness	Rock Water

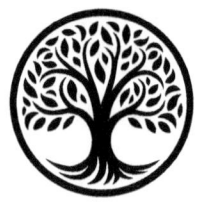

"Our sorrows and wounds are healed only when we touch them with compassion."

— BUDDHA

CHAPTER 7

Bodywork

Touch is one of the oldest and most natural forms of healing. While bodywork alone might not fully resolve anxiety, it pairs well with many other approaches I'll be sharing. Using these methods together can provide long-term support for managing anxiety. What they all have in common is the power of human connection through touch. The simple, compassionate touch from another person can bring immediate comfort, even without any prior relationship. Research shows that premature babies who receive gentle touch, hugs, or stroking tend to gain weight faster than those who don't. Practitioners skilled in touch therapies, such as massage, reflexology, or Reiki, have a unique gift. From my own experiences, I've always felt that they bring a unique, caring energy that truly supports healing.

Massage

If you haven't tried a massage yet, now's a great time to give it a go! Massage is one of the oldest healing practices, with records going back about 4,000 years in China. Since your skin is the largest organ in your body, massage is designed to activate your body's natural ability to heal and restore balance. It works quickly, making it especially helpful on stressful days. Massage calms and refreshes your nervous system, relieves muscle and joint pain, and boosts circulation to help nourish your whole body.

I get that massages can sometimes feel like a luxury or might not always fit into your schedule or budget, but even a short session can do wonders for relaxation and easing anxiety. Many places offer quick, affordable ten-minute chair massages that are surprisingly effective. It's also worth checking with your health insurance to see if massage therapy is covered.

Reflexology

Reflexology entails applying pressure to specific points on the hands or feet, which correspond to the body's internal systems and organs. Tailoring the approach to address specific concerns, whether it's back or neck pain, kidney or liver issues, the reflexologist targets these points to increase circulation and initiate the body's innate healing processes. For alleviating anxiety, particular attention is given to the solar plexus reflex (stomach area), where anxiety is often most pronounced. The treatment then extends to every reflex, restoring natural balance and harmony. The positive calming effects persist even after the session concludes. Reflexology, especially when combined with essential oils during treatment, is a wonderful experience.

Reiki

Reiki, a healing method originating in Japan, was developed by Dr. Mikao Usui in the early 20th century. The term "Reiki" is derived from two Japanese words: "rei," which signifies spiritual or higher power consciousness, and "ki," similar to "chi" in Chinese or "prana" in Hindu, representing life energy or the universal life force. While not a religion, Reiki holds spiritual significance. The higher power or consciousness, called Rei, guides the life energy, known as ki, in what is known as Reiki. The underlying principle of Reiki is the belief that all living things possess universal life energy, and practitioners can channel this energy to facilitate healing, relaxation, and overall well-being.

The concept suggests that maintaining a balance in life energy is crucial, as depletion makes one susceptible to illness. Ki, the essence of our emotions, thoughts, and spiritual life, is everywhere and can be consciously accumulated and directed.

During a Reiki session, the practitioner uses their hands to lightly touch or hover over and scan the body, focusing on specific areas with potential energy blockages. The goal is to balance and strengthen the body's energy flow. Interestingly, issues in one part of the body may originate from elsewhere. Practitioners act as conduits for Reiki, allowing the energy to flow through them to the recipient.

Reiki is accessible to everyone but channeling it to others requires an attunement from a Reiki Master. Those attuned can even perform Reiki on themselves. This practice has shown remarkable results in alleviating anxiety and depression. References for practitioners and classes are listed at the end of the book.

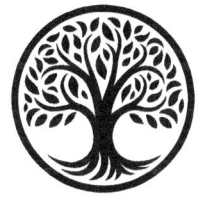

> "Feelings come and go like clouds in a windy sky. Conscious breathing is my anchor."
>
> — Thich Nhat Hanh

CHAPTER 8

Breathing

Breathing is one of the simplest, most accessible tools we have for managing anxiety, yet it's often overlooked. When anxiety hits, our breath tends to become shallow and rapid, feeding the body's stress response and intensifying feelings of panic or overwhelm. But by slowing down and breathing deeply, we can begin to shift our internal state almost instantly.

Deep, intentional breaths activate the parasympathetic nervous system, which is our body's natural "rest and restore" mode. This helps to counteract the fight-or-flight response triggered by anxiety, calming the mind, lowering stress hormones like cortisol, and steadying a racing heart. In just a few moments, you can transition from chaos to calm by simply tuning into the breath.

Bringing attention to your breath grounds you in the present moment. It anchors the mind and interrupts the spiral of anxious thoughts. This mindful awareness creates space to pause and engage with the moment more calmly.

Beyond the immediate calming effects, deep breathing also enhances oxygen flow to the brain and vital organs. Over time, this improved oxygenation supports clearer thinking, emotional balance, and overall resilience. In the midst of life's noise and demands, the breath offers a quiet refuge, a simple, steady rhythm that's always with you, waiting to bring you back to center.

Let's begin with Alternate Nostril Breathing. This is my favorite breathing technique. It's incredibly simple, and you can practice it anytime you feel overwhelmed and need to find your center.

Alternate Nostril Breathing

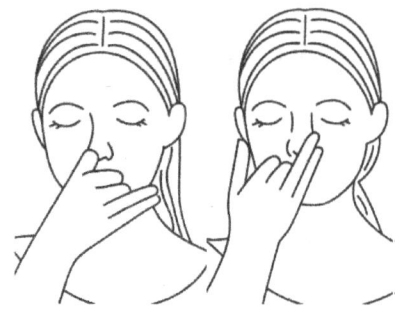

1. Use your right thumb to close your right nostril gently. Inhale slowly through your left nostril for a count of four seconds.

2. Then, close your left nostril with your right ring and little finger, release your right thumb from the right nostril, and exhale slowly through the right nostril for a count of eight seconds. This completes half a round.

3. Next, inhale through the right nostril for four seconds. Close the right nostril with your right thumb again, release the left nostril, and exhale through the left nostril for eight seconds. This completes one full round.

Start with a few rounds twice a day and work up to five minutes a day.

CAUTION: Avoid practicing alternate nostril breathing if you have a cold or if your nasal passages are blocked. Forcing breath through obstructed nostrils can lead to complications. Never force anything. If you're using your nostrils for breath control, ensure they are unobstructed.

The 4-7-8 Breath

This simple breathing technique is great for calming anxiety or managing an anxiety attack, and you can do it discreetly anywhere.

Start by gently placing the tip of your tongue against the ridge just behind your upper front teeth and keep it there throughout the exercise. You'll be exhaling quietly through your mouth around your tongue. Focus on breathing deeply from your belly.

The important part is to make your exhale twice as long as your inhale. This longer exhale helps your body relax and ease tension.

- Exhale completely through your mouth.
- Close your mouth and inhale through your nose to a mental count of four.
- Hold your breath for a count of seven.
- Exhale completely through your mouth to a count of eight. This is one breath. Repeat the cycle three more times for a total of four breaths.

Since your exhale lasts twice as long as your inhale, it may feel uncomfortable at first; however, with consistent practice, you'll notice deeper breathing patterns. When I first attempted this, I experienced mild lightheadedness, but it faded quickly. If you feel lightheaded, pause before continuing. If the sensation persists, stop.

For the first month, limit yourself to no more than four rounds. Over time, you can gradually increase the repetitions. I've found this exercise to have a lasting impact. Even after finishing, you will continue to feel the positive effects.

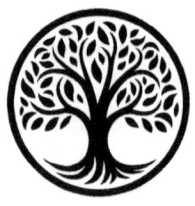

> "There are no worthless herbs, only the lack of knowledge."
>
> — AVICENNA

CHAPTER 9

CBD aka Cannabidiol

I'm fortunate to be connected to a diverse network of skilled practitioners and amazing healers. Among them, Dori Bell stands out for her deep expertise in CBD, and I'm truly grateful for her generosity in sharing her knowledge and contributing as an author to this work.

Dori's Biography

Dori Bell is a certified aromatherapist and cannabis practitioner specializing in combining the power of essential oils with CBD for the best wellness outcome for her clients. She has received the CIBTAC-endorsed LabCannamist training and certification for working with cannabis and CBD therapeutically and has been practicing aromatherapy professionally since 2000.

Read more about her and her work at **www.theblossombar.com**.

CBD: Your Ally Against Anxiety

By Dori Bell

CBD is a natural way to combat anxiety and a powerful tool to have on hand during times of stress. In my practice, I've seen clients regain their peace of mind and feel more like themselves than they have in years, thanks to CBD.

A lot of misinformation exists on CBD and its parent plant, *Cannabis sativa*. Here, you'll learn what CBD is, how it works in the body, and what makes it so effective against anxiety. As a CBD-certified aromatherapist with over twenty years of experience, I incorporate essential oils and natural companions to CBD that enhance its effectiveness in the body.

What is CBD?

CBD is short for cannabidiol, an organic chemical compound found in the *Cannabis sativa* plant. It is one of the non-psychoactive phytocannabinoids found in cannabis and hemp plants, meaning it does not intoxicate like THC (tetrahydrocannabinol), another phytocannabinoid, does.

Most CBD on the market is extracted from hemp, which is simply *Cannabis sativa* containing less than 0.3% THC in its chemical makeup.

Increasing amounts of research and studies are showing that CBD has anxiolytic (anti-anxiety) properties, decreasing anxiety while increasing mental sedation. Let's look at how this works.

How It Works in the Body on Anxiety

CBD interacts with brain receptors that regulate fear and anxiety through indirect interaction with neurotransmitters like serotonin and dopamine. It does this by indirectly impacting our endocannabinoid system (ECS).

Our ECS is crucial to the process because it interacts with multiple body systems, including the immune, nervous, and digestive systems. The ECS helps the body adapt to stressors by promoting balance and homeostasis. One of its vital functions is its ability to override our fight-or-flight response so that we don't experience unnecessary amounts of cortisol, the "stress hormone." CBD influences specific serotonin receptors to make serotonin more available in the brain. The more serotonin our bodies have on hand to work with, the quicker harmony within our bodies can be reestablished.

CBD Guidelines

Knowing which CBD to buy and in which form to buy it can be confusing. The best course of action is to work with a certified cannabis practitioner to determine the correct dosing of CBD for you.

First, decide how you will administer the CBD: topically or orally.

- Topically is a good option if anxiety has resulted in muscle aches and stiffness, and if you want the CBD to take longer to impact.
- Orally is a good option to get the CBD into the bloodstream quickly, to manage ongoing anxiety, and for times of active anxiety.

Next, decide which form to buy the CBD in whether a liquid tincture or an edible food product. Note that CBD is often referred to as "hemp extract" on the label and product description.

You'll have three options when purchasing a CBD tincture:

- **CBD Full Spectrum** is an extract of the full *Cannabis sativa* plant and may contain THC. This form of CBD is not legal in some places, and a medical card may be required to purchase it.

- **CBD Broad Spectrum** is extracted from the full plant but goes through an additional process to remove the THC and contains less than 0.3% THC. This form of CBD is the most common. It is sometimes called CBD distillate.
- **CBD Isolate** contains 0% THC. It contains only CBD. This option may be harder to find, but it should be available at most dispensaries or even drugstores in some countries and U.S. states.

Reputable distributors will have the certificate of analysis (COA) readily available for each CBD product on their websites. The COA will tell you the concentration of CBD in the product and the percentage of THC (if any) present in the product.

NOTE: Hempseed oil is not CBD. Unscrupulous companies will sell hempseed oil and call it CBD or hemp extract. It is neither of those things. It is a beautiful and nutrient-dense carrier oil often used in skin care products and aromatherapy.

Edibles are fun and convenient, but notoriously inconsistent with how much CBD you're getting in each bite. If you are sensitive or just starting your CBD journey, I'd recommend getting to know how your body reacts to it with a tincture, with which you can carefully control the dose.

CBD tincture comes in different concentrations. The concentration will determine the potency of each drop of CBD tincture. For someone new to CBD, I recommend starting with the lowest concentration and observing how your body responds.

The number one rule for CBD dosing is "low and slow." Anxiety, in particular, responds best to low and consistent oral dosing of CBD tincture. Start with a low potency and fewer drops throughout the day and gradually increase the dosage until you reach the desired level.

Generally, start with two drops of CBD tincture (this is usually 2 mg) under the tongue three times per day around meals, increasing by one drop per day until you feel the anxiety lessen and become more manageable. Note how you feel in a journal.

I've seen my more sensitive clients experience dizziness and nausea using low doses of broad-spectrum CBD. You may want to start with CBD isolate and work your way up to broad-spectrum if you're sensitive to medications.

Another important dosing rule is to stop CBD two hours before bedtime for the most restful sleep.

IMPORTANT NOTE: Let your doctor know you plan on adding CBD to your routine if you are taking anti-anxiety medication or antidepressants.

Role of Terpenes and the Entourage Effect

Terpenes are the most common class of organic compounds found in plants that give them their color, taste, aroma, and many of their therapeutic properties. The terpenes in *Cannabis sativa* enhance the effects of the cannabinoids (such as CBD and THC) within it, most notably their ability to manage anxiety.

Many of the important terpenes in the cannabis plant are removed during the CBD extraction process, making CBD less terpene-rich than the full plant and therefore less effective against anxiety. A theory called the Entourage Effect, briefly summarized as the whole cannabis plant working synergistically to produce the most optimal result, explains that having even that .3% THC in a CBD product improves its efficacy and why full-spectrum and THC-containing cannabis, full of terpene goodness, works best of all.

If you don't want the THC or only want broad-spectrum CBD, there is an option to boost the terpene content and therefore the efficacy of a topical CBD application: high-terpene essential oils.

Anxiety, Essential Oils, and CBD

Essential oils have been used for thousands of years because they can positively impact our well-being. Due to their molecular makeup, many essential oils help the body manage and recover from anxiety in a pleasant and enjoyable way.

Essential oils contain terpenes just like cannabis does, and these terpenes can fill in for the terpenes that have been removed in the CBD extraction process. This allows the Entourage Effect to work its magic without the intoxication of THC and with the added enjoyment of the fragrance of the essential oils.

It's important to note here that essential oils have powerful effects in the body, just as CBD does. There are complementary relationships and intricacies at work within the essential oils, and each person's chemical makeup and past experiences must be considered before an essential oil recommendation is made. Working with a certified, experienced aromatherapist is always recommended for optimal and safe results.

How to Use Essential Oils with CBD

Combine the essential oils with your CBD tincture in a carrier oil, such as fractionated coconut oil or jojoba, to create a massage blend that helps the body manage and recover from anxiety.

Ingesting essential oils is generally not a safe practice and should only be done under the guidance of a certified clinical aromatherapist.

High-Terpene Essential Oils for Anxiety

Essential oils with high percentages of monoterpenes, sesquiterpenes, and monoterpenols help CBD work most effectively in the body and have their own anti-anxiety properties.

Some to consider are:

- Coriander *(Coriandrum sativum L.)*
- Geranium *(Pelargonium graveolens)*
- Lavender *(Lavandula angustifolia)*
- Lime *(Citrus aurantifolia)*
- Neroli *(Citrus aurantium var. amara)*
- Orange *(Citrus sinensis)*
- Palo Santo *(Bursera graveolens)*
- Patchouli *(Pogostemon cablin)*
- Pine *(Pinus sylvestris)*
- Ylang Ylang *(Cananga odorata)*

CBD is a powerful ally against anxiety. It can help you manage and reduce the symptoms of anxiety and help harmonize your body. With a more balanced and calm nervous system, you are more likely to have the internal space to identify the root cause of the anxiety. Adding essential oils to topical applications of CBD brings even more therapeutic power into the mix.

CBD helps with more than just anxiety, too. It can help ease chronic pain, digestive issues, inflammation, migraines, epilepsy, and autoimmune diseases.

One final consideration as you begin your CBD journey: CBD is not for everyone. Allergic reactions to *Cannabis sativa* and, hence, CBD are possible, as with any plant. Those highly sensitive to medications and supplements, and those working to wean themselves off antidepressants, may experience dizziness and nausea. If in doubt, ask your doctor and work with, ideally, a cannabis-trained aromatherapist.

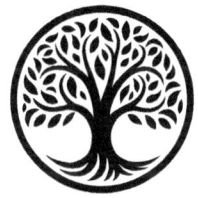

> "When the diet is wrong, medicine is of no use. When diet is correct, medicine is of no need."
>
> — Ayurvedic Proverb

CHAPTER 10

Diet

Despite the abundance of information available on diet and nutrition, there's still not enough emphasis on just how crucial our dietary choices are to overall health, especially their direct link to anxiety. Diet isn't just about maintaining a healthy weight; it significantly influences mood, behavior, and mental clarity. This food–mood connection is an often-overlooked aspect of emotional well-being. What we eat affects how we feel, think, and respond to stress, making nutrition an essential tool in supporting mental and emotional health.

Take sugar, for example. Overconsumption, particularly in children, can trigger behavioral changes like hyperactivity or aggression. Stabilizing blood sugar levels can help regulate mood and improve both emotional and mental well-being.

One of the biggest dietary culprits? Ultra-processed foods. These foods undergo heavy industrial processing and often contain a cocktail of additives, including preservatives, artificial colors and flavors, emulsifiers, and sweeteners.

They're typically low in nutrients and high in refined sugars, unhealthy fats, and sodium. Think of sugary drinks, packaged snacks, fast food, and even many cereals and yogurts marketed as "healthy." Unless you're buying plain yogurt and cereals, they're likely loaded with sugar.

In fairness, parents are not taught how to read nutrition labels or provided basic guidance on food quality when raising a child. According to the U.S. National Institutes of Health, ultra-processed foods may disrupt hunger hormones, leading to increased cravings and overeating past the point of fullness, which can result in weight gain and related health concerns.

The good news is that awareness is growing. More people are becoming educated about the hidden ingredients in our food supply and the profound connection between what we eat and how we feel, mentally and emotionally.

As we'll explore further in the next chapter, a diet that supports gut health can play a powerful role in reducing anxiety. Fiber-rich and fermented foods, such as kefir, plain yogurt, and sauerkraut nourish beneficial gut bacteria, which support both digestion and emotional stability. For those who are lactose intolerant or avoid dairy, non-dairy probiotic options, such as coconut or almond yogurt, are excellent alternatives.

So, What Does an Anxiety-Friendly Diet Look Like?

It starts with whole, unprocessed foods, colorful fruits and vegetables, whole grains, nuts, seeds, and high-quality proteins like wild salmon, beans, and grass-fed, grass-finished meats. When choosing poultry or pork, seek out humanely raised, pasture-fed sources.

Remember, meat shouldn't dominate your plate. Think of it as a condiment. Center your meals around plant-based foods for more stable energy and improved mood.

Avoid refined carbohydrates such as white sugar, flour, and rice. These high-glycemic foods cause blood sugar spikes and crashes that can worsen anxiety symptoms, and if the body doesn't utilize this excess blood sugar, it is stored as fat.

Instead, opt for 100% whole-grain or gluten-free alternatives that provide sustained energy release. Great options include farro, barley, bulgur, quinoa, brown rice, oats, and buckwheat.

Diets high in caffeine, sugar, and processed foods have consistently been linked to higher anxiety levels. On the flip side, eating more whole foods such as fresh fruits, vegetables, and plenty of fiber can help you feel more balanced and emotionally steady.

One of the most researched and effective dietary approaches is the Mediterranean diet, which emphasizes whole foods and healthy fats. Studies show that people who follow this lifestyle tend to have lower anxiety levels than those eating a typical Western diet high in sugar and processed ingredients.

Additionally, research suggests that omega-3 fatty acids, found in fatty fish, flaxseeds, and walnuts, offer mental health benefits. These nutrients not only support brain health but are also associated with reduced anxiety and inflammation.

The takeaway? You are what you eat, emotionally, mentally, and physically.

> **READ LABELS!** Avoid artificial sweeteners, partially hydrogenated oils, and high-fructose corn syrup. Monitor your salt intake as it can elevate blood pressure and deplete the body of essential potassium, which is crucial for a healthy nervous system. If you can't identify an ingredient on a food label, don't buy it.

As mentioned earlier, caffeine exacerbates anxiety. Consider switching to decaf, herbal tea, or a coffee substitute, such as Teeccino. It consists of a blend of herbs, grains, fruits, and nuts, which also benefits digestive health.

Don't Forget About Water!

Staying well-hydrated is key to keeping your brain sharp and your anxiety in check. While everyone's needs vary based on age, body size, activity level, and even the weather, a general guideline is to aim for approximately eight cups of water per day, which is roughly 64 ounces or 2 liters. But hydration isn't one-size-fits-all.

As we age, our sense of thirst naturally diminishes, making it easier to become dehydrated without realizing it. Proper hydration is essential for maintaining brain function, supporting joint health, aiding digestion, and sustaining energy. Chronic dehydration can lead to confusion, constipation, urinary tract infections, kidney problems, and even an increased risk of falls. The decline in thirst sensation typically begins around age 60, but changes can start as early as the mid-50s for some people.

The best advice? Listen to your body. If you're thirsty, drink! Other signs you might be dehydrated include a dry mouth, low energy, dizziness, or dark yellow urine. And if you're exercising in a hot climate or feeling under the weather, your body will need even more fluids to compensate for the loss of fluids through sweat and breathing. Maintaining a healthy water intake is a simple yet effective way to support both physical and emotional well-being.

Foods that are good for anxiety include:
- Apricots
- Asparagus
- Avocado (high in fat - but good fat)
- Bananas
- Beans
- Broccoli
- Brown rice and whole grains

- Dried Fruit
- Figs
- Fish (especially wild Alaskan salmon)
- Garlic
- Green leafy vegetables
- Raw nuts and seeds
- Plain yogurt – preferably organic

These foods supply minerals such as calcium, magnesium, phosphorus, and potassium, which are depleted by stress. Not only will these diet recommendations help your anxiety, but they are also great for your overall health.

It's important to note that while diet can significantly impact anxiety, it's not a standalone solution. It works best in conjunction with other lifestyle changes.

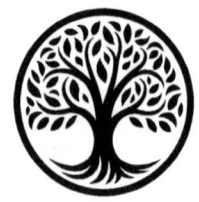

> "All disease begins in the gut."
>
> — HIPPOCRATES

CHAPTER 11

Digestive Health

Your digestive system isn't just about breaking down food. It's home to trillions of tiny organisms like bacteria, fungi, and even viruses. Together, they make up what's called your gut microbiome. Think of it as a microscopic community that helps run key parts of your body.

This gut crew does way more than help you digest. It supports your immune system, helps manage metabolism, produces certain vitamins, and even affects your mood and mental health. When things get out of balance, something called gut dysbiosis can lead to a bunch of issues, including anxiety.

So, keeping your gut microbiome happy and balanced isn't just about digestion, it's a key part of your overall health.

Lately, there's been a lot of discussion around how your gut health is tied to your mental health, especially when it comes to things like anxiety. It turns out your gut and brain are in constant conversation through something called the gut-brain axis, a two-way communication system that links your digestive system with your nervous system.

This connection is a big deal. It involves your gut microbes, your brain, and even your hormones, all working together to influence your mood, stress levels, and how you handle anxiety.

Around 90 to 95% of your serotonin, which is the feel-good hormone that helps stabilize mood, is made in your gut, not your brain. Therefore, when your digestive system is acting up, it can impact your emotional well-being.

This mind-body connection is far from a new concept. Ancient healing traditions, such as Ayurveda and Traditional Chinese Medicine, have long recognized that maintaining digestive health is crucial to overall mental and emotional well-being.

While medications and supplements can help alleviate conditions like GERD and bloating, they are temporary solutions. They address the symptoms without tackling the underlying causes, such as what you eat and what occupies your thoughts and emotions. Quick fixes might seem helpful in the moment, but they can lead to bigger problems down the line, especially when it comes to your digestive and mental health. Your brain and digestive system are constantly in communication, and when that balance is disrupted, it can impact your immune response, nervous system, and even your mood.

The body is surprisingly intuitive. We often experience emotions physically, such as the instinctive "gut feeling" or the "butterflies" in your stomach when you're nervous. These sensations aren't just figures of speech; they're signs of the strong connection between your digestive system and your brain.

Probiotics can be helpful in certain situations, but it's important to consult your healthcare provider before starting them. They can help you choose the right strain, as different strains serve different purposes, and advise on the best timing, especially if you're taking antibiotics, to avoid any potential interactions. While probiotics are often promoted as essential for gut health, the scientific evidence supporting their everyday use is still limited and evolving.

Some studies suggest that they might help reduce anxiety by supporting the microbiome, but the most reliable way to improve gut health remains straightforward. Maintain a fiber-rich, balanced diet and adopt a healthy lifestyle that incorporates regular exercise, effective stress management, social connections, and a sense of purpose. In the end, there's no magic pill, just good nutrition, smart habits, and paying attention to what your body needs.

A diet rich in various high-fiber plants, nuts, and fermented foods helps maintain a range of beneficial bacteria in the gut. The more varied your diet, the more diverse your microbiome, which is associated with better overall health. Fiber serves as food for these beneficial gut bacteria, promoting a healthy microbial environment and enhancing digestion. It can also help reduce the risk of various gut-related conditions.

Herbal teas, such as marshmallow and slippery elm, can also help heal the digestive tract. In Ayurveda, we use an herb known as Triphala. Its name translates to "three fruits," comprising a combination of three fruits native to the Indian subcontinent: Amalaki, Bibhitaki, and Haritaki. The synergistic effect of these three fruits yields powerful benefits within the body. Triphala is a potent antioxidant that supports digestion and acts as a natural, gentle laxative. Additionally, it contributes to the well-being of the nervous, cardiovascular, respiratory, and reproductive systems and can aid in weight loss.

- **Amalaki** (*Emblica officinalis* or Indian gooseberry) is known for its high vitamin C and antioxidant content, supports the immune system, and promotes overall health.
- **Bibhitaki** (*Terminalia bellirica*) has astringent properties and supports respiratory health, digestion, and detoxification.

- **Haritaki** (*Terminalia chebula*) has laxative and detoxifying effects. It's also considered beneficial for digestive health and can support the removal of toxins from the body.

You also have the option to acquire an at-home test kit from companies such as Viome, Thorn, Function Health, and Standard Process to assess your microbiome. These tests are diagnostic assessments that analyze the composition of bacteria, fungi, viruses, and other microorganisms in an individual's gastrointestinal tract. It typically involves collecting a stool sample and using various techniques, such as DNA sequencing, to identify and quantify the microorganisms present. The results of these tests can provide valuable insights into the diversity, balance, and overall health of the gut microbiome. You will receive personalized insights and recommendations to improve your gut health. However, a functional medicine doctor can help decipher the test results and devise a personalized nutritional plan tailored to your unique bio-individuality.

The journey to healing the gut is a gradual process, especially if you have been ignoring symptoms or relying on antacids. A good starting point is eliminating sugar, dairy, and gluten from your diet for two to three months. Increase your intake of fruits and vegetables and opt for organic options whenever possible. If you eat meat, opt for grass-fed, grass-finished, and pasture-raised options that are free from antibiotics. Finding a functional medicine doctor, a registered dietitian, a nutritionist, or a certified health coach to work with can be helpful.

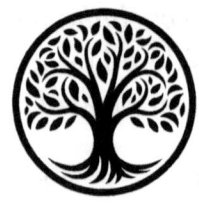

"Incredible things can be done simply if we are committed to making them happen."

— Sadhguru

CHAPTER 12

Emotional Freedom Technique

Marian Buck-Murray is another of the outstanding practitioners I have had the privilege to know. I'm deeply grateful that she agreed to share her insights and expertise on Emotional Freedom Technique (EFT). Her wisdom and guidance have been invaluable, and I'm excited to have the opportunity to learn from her and pass along her knowledge.

Marian's Biography

Marian Buck-Murray is a Certified EFT Practitioner and Matrix Reimprinting Practitioner. She specializes in helping sensitive and creative people step out of the shadows. Visit her website at www.marianbuckmurray.com for videos on how to use EFT Tapping or connect with her on Instagram @MarianBuckMurray.

EFT Tapping — An Easy-to-Use Tool to Release Anxiety

By Marian Buck-Murray

Emotional Freedom Techniques, also known as EFT and Tapping, is an evidence-based acupressure tapping technique in which participants use their fingers to tap specific acupressure points on the hands, torso, and face. Based on Chinese acupuncture, EFT helps clear energy disruptions and calm the nervous system. EFT is used to neutralize uncomfortable feelings such as anxiety, sadness, anger, and more. The basic tapping routine is easy to use and memorize.

Randomized controlled studies have demonstrated EFT's ability to significantly reduce the stress hormone cortisol. Because tapping reduces cortisol, it is a highly effective tool for anxiety. High cortisol and anxiety go hand in hand. When cortisol is reduced, so is anxiety, and vice versa. Simply tapping on the side of the hand is enough to begin reducing both cortisol and anxiety.

EFT has been extensively investigated for both anxiety and depression. In a large-scale study of 5,000 patients seeking treatment for anxiety, improvement was found in 90% of patients who received acupressure tapping therapy compared to 63% of the Cognitive Behavior Therapy participants.

EFT can be used with a certified practitioner and as a self-help technique. Certified EFT Practitioners are trained to help clients resolve triggers, emotions, negative beliefs, physical pain, trauma, and behavior patterns. Often, a client will benefit the most from the support of a compassionate, certified professional. Additionally, there are numerous ways to utilize EFT as a quick and effective self-help technique. The most common and straightforward formula for EFT Tapping is simple.

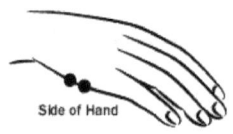
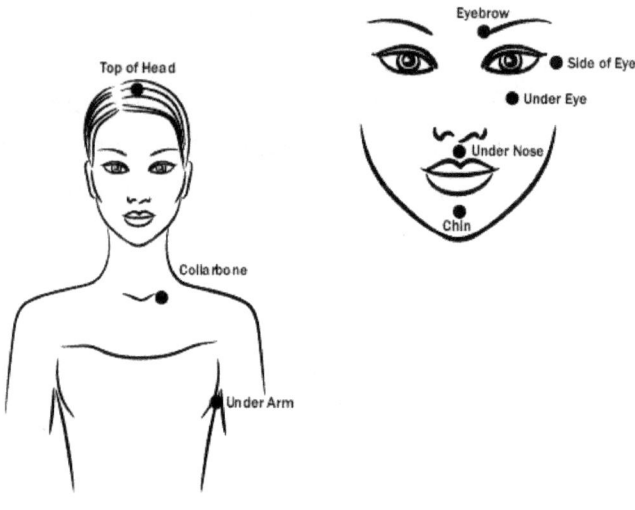

Illustration courtesy of Thomas Murray

EFT Tapping Points

While using the basic recipe, it's important to consider a specific feeling or triggering circumstance. This is referred to as the target or problem. Notice where and how it feels in your body and determine the intensity of the feeling. While focusing on this feeling, tap on the acupressure points while saying phrases that describe the feeling and/or triggering circumstance. The tapping sequence will help neutralize the feeling.

After each round of tapping, tune in to assess any changes in intensity or body sensations. One round of tapping is usually enough to help calm the nervous system and reduce some intensity. Additional rounds of tapping will help reduce the feeling further or even eliminate it.

CASE STUDIES:
EFT's Applications in Reducing Anxiety

Woman in Class: Many years ago, I was teaching a public class when I saw that a woman in the front row was experiencing feelings of panic. She was out of her seat, ready to leave the class. Not wanting her to leave in such a panicked state, I showed her how to tap on the side of her hand while breathing deeply. After just a few moments, she was able to relax back in her chair and stay for the rest of the class.

Client Speaking Up at a Business Meeting: A client expressed exasperation with her difficulty speaking up at business meetings. I explained to her that anxiety triggers high cortisol, which triggers blood loss from the thinking part of the brain. This includes the part that helps us articulate clearly. EFT helps reduce cortisol, allowing blood to return to the brain and making speaking much easier. We tapped on her feelings of anxiety, using her visceral sense of a typical business meeting as our target. I also recommended that she tap on the side of her hand, under the table, if necessary, before speaking. Both techniques helped her speak up and articulate her thoughts clearly.

Singing in Front of People: One client came to me frustrated with her inability to follow through with her desire to sing in public. She told me that the thought of it made her shrink into panic mode. Although she knew she had a beautiful singing voice, she couldn't muster the courage to go further. In our work together, we uncovered a childhood situation in which she was ridiculed for her singing. Using this situation as the target, we helped reduce the intensity of the feeling. Continuing this tapping on her own, she was able to eliminate nearly all of the anxiety. She now creates and sings in her own shows.

How to Use EFT Tapping as a Self-Help Technique

Tapping in the Moment

Tapping on the side of the hand while breathing deeply is enough to help reduce feelings of panic and anxiety. The deep breath activates the relaxation response, while the tapping calms your nervous system.

Tapping for a Future Event

Anxiety can be all-consuming when we're faced with a future event, such as a party, interview, business meeting, or romantic date. Using the basic EFT recipe while tuning into the anxiety and imagining the future event will help neutralize the anxiety. Repeating this process will continue to reduce any remaining anxiety. Once the anxiety feels manageable, it's helpful to tap and repeat positive, encouraging phrases to boost confidence.

Rant and Tap to Release the Day's Anxieties

Anxiety and high cortisol can interfere with a good night's sleep. The Rant and Tap technique is an effective way to calm the nervous system before bed. Tap on all of the points while ranting about the day's events. Tap for as long as needed. This tapping technique will help reduce cortisol levels and clear the mind.

Tapping with the Feeling as a Target

When you experience anxiety or panic, pause to focus on how it feels in your body. Tap through the points, breathing deeply without speaking a word. Simply tap and focus on the feeling. Continue tapping until the feeling becomes manageable or is completely neutralized.

Though EFT Tapping has numerous far-reaching applications, it is especially effective for anxiety. Among the types of anxiety it helps are performance anxiety, sports anxiety, dental care anxiety, medical anxiety, test anxiety, social anxiety, and just about every other kind of anxiety. Best of all, it's simple to use and right at your fingertips.

The EFT (Emotional Freedom Techniques) Basic Recipe:

1. **Choose a specific problem, issue, or event.**
   Notice where you feel it in your body.

2. **Rate the intensity of the feeling on a scale of 0-10**
   (0 being the least intense and 10 being the most).

3. **Create a setup statement.**
   Name your problem, issue, or event. Create a set-up statement: "Even though I have this [problem], I completely accept myself."

4. **Create a reminder phrase to describe your problem.**
   You can use one reminder phrase for the entire sequence or a variety of phrases that tap into the same problem. When beginning, it's easiest to use one reminder phrase, such as "this anxiety." The reminder phrase can be the same as the problem in the setup statement.

5. **Use a setup phrase on the side of the hand point.**
   Repeat the set-up statement three times while tapping on the side of the hand point.

6. **Use the reminder phrase while tapping on each of the following points:**
   - Eyebrow Point
   - Side of Eye
   - Under Eye
   - Under Nose

- Chin
- Collarbone
- Under Arms
- Top of Head

7. **Reassess after the sequence**

   Determine the intensity level of the feeling.

8. **Repeat the sequence until the intensity is at 2 or lower.**

   Vary the phrasing of the set-up statement and reminder phrase as the problem shifts. For example, you might say, *"This remaining [problem]."*

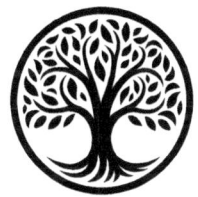

> "When you dance, your purpose is not to get to a certain place on the floor; it's to enjoy each step along the way."
>
> — Dr. Wayne Dyer

CHAPTER 13

Exercise

Extensive research now confirms that regular physical activity can not only alleviate anxiety but also potentially prevent it. Further studies have shown that exercise can be as effective as antidepressant medications in treating depression and preventing relapses. Exercise has a profoundly positive effect on mental, emotional, and physical well-being.

The mechanism behind this lies in the release of endorphins, which are natural brain chemicals that act as pain and stress relievers. Research from Johns Hopkins University indicates that moderately intense activities yield the most significant benefits. It's important to remember that you don't have to be drenched in sweat to get meaningful results. Gentle, steady activities like walking, swimming, dancing, biking, or yoga can be incredibly effective. In contrast, competitive sports, while fun for some, can add more stress, which isn't always helpful when you're trying to support your nervous system.

Incorporating mind-body practices, such as yoga and tai chi, can further calm the mind and boost energy levels. The key is to engage in safe and enjoyable activities that shift focus away from anxiety. I've outlined a few types of exercises that are highly beneficial.

Walking

A study at the University of Texas at Austin revealed that just thirty minutes of brisk walking on a treadmill surpasses resting in generating feelings of well-being and increasing energy levels. Participants in the study reported reduced levels of anxiety, depression, anger, and fatigue after walking. The positive effects of exercise were nearly instantaneous, and mood improved immediately following the treadmill session, remaining elevated for up to an hour.

If time is a constraint, research indicates that even short bursts of exercise can be remarkably beneficial, especially as a starting point. You don't need an elaborate gym or expensive equipment to get a great workout. Sometimes, a simple walk can work wonders. I make it a point to walk outside daily whenever the weather allows, and I use my treadmill on days when that's not possible. Walking in nature provides a much-needed break from the hustle and bustle of daily life. Knowing that I'm prioritizing my health keeps me motivated to stay committed to my goals.

Brisk walking offers essential aerobic benefits for overall health. Dr. Andrew Weil recommends aiming to cover three miles in about forty-five minutes, a goal you can work towards gradually. Walking is a fantastic way to connect with nature, reduce stress, and improve your well-being, all in one activity!

Yoga

I've practiced and taught yoga for many years, and I know firsthand how powerful it can be. On stressful days, I consistently feel calmer and more balanced after a session. Yoga fosters presence and mindfulness, guiding attention away from anxious thoughts. Through focused movement and breathwork, it creates a sense of calm, grounding, and inner clarity.

As your practice deepens, the effects are cumulative. It will help you cope better with issues ranging from grief to road rage. As you become more aware, you are better equipped to put things into clearer perspective. It will help you get to the bottom of your anxiety.

A study from the University of Brazil involved fourteen volunteers who suffered from anxiety participating in yoga classes. After one month, there was a significant reduction in anxiety, depression, and tension, as well as an increase in well-being.

Practicing yoga even a few times a week will enhance your well-being. It teaches us to pause and increase patience and compassion. In the process, we also become more comfortable and familiar with our bodies. This leads to greater self-confidence, which helps us control our thoughts.

Tai Chi

Tai Chi originated in China over 3,000 years ago and is a traditional Chinese martial art often referred to as "meditation in motion." Its healing power comes from the combination of slow, fluid movements focusing on relaxation, balance, and mindfulness. These graceful movements enhance the flow of chi (life energy) throughout the body, improving strength, balance, flexibility, and concentration. Additionally, Tai Chi enhances blood circulation and strengthens the immune system, making it an ideal practice that nurtures both body and mind.

Tai Chi is suitable for people of all ages and fitness levels and can be practiced both indoors and outdoors. Its gentle nature makes it particularly beneficial for older adults or those with physical limitations.

Keep It Fun and Social

Exercising with someone is a great way to stay motivated. Don't forget that gardening, swimming, biking, golfing, bowling, using the stairs when you can, and dancing (even alone in your room) are all fun, beneficial forms of exercise. Try something new! How about a belly dancing class or jumping on a trampoline? The idea is to move your body, free your mind, release endorphins, and work off that stress. Keep it fun!

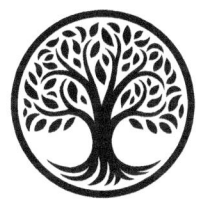

"Parsley, sage, rosemary, and thyme...."

— SIMON & GARFUNKEL

CHAPTER 14

Herbs

Nature offers a pharmacy for nearly every condition. For thousands of years, herbs have been used to support the body's natural ability to heal by strengthening the immune system. As an herbalist, I often recommend herbs for managing anxiety and depression.

Herbs are available in various forms, including pills, capsules, teas, and tinctures. Tinctures are liquid herbal extracts stored in dark glass bottles with droppers, making it easy to add a few drops to water or juice. While incorporating herbs into your daily diet can provide nutritional support, addressing specific health concerns may require larger or more targeted doses. Some herbs provide fast relief, while others work more gradually, with their full benefits building over time.

Even the most experienced herbalists will tell you there's no one-size-fits-all solution. Each person's needs are different, and it often takes some trial and error with various herbs and dosages to find what works best for you. Working with a qualified herbalist can help you determine which herbs are best suited to your unique needs.

Nervines

Nervines are herbs that impact the nervous system, which include the brain, spinal cord, and a network of nerves responsible for transmitting messages between the brain and the body. Supporting the nervous system, in turn, benefits other systems such as the immune, cardiovascular, adrenal, and digestive systems.

Nervines can help calm the body and soothe a stressed or anxious mind. They fall into three categories: nervine tonics, nervine relaxants, and nervine stimulants. For managing anxiety, I'll focus on relaxants and tonics. Relaxants have a calming effect, while tonics nourish and support the central nervous system. These herbs boost GABA in the brain to calm the nervous system and ease anxiety, much like certain pharmaceuticals but usually without their side effects.

Below are some of my favorite nervines, which can be taken in tea, pill, or tincture form.

Lavender (Lavandula angustifolia)

Many clinical studies have been conducted on the effectiveness of lavender for anxiety and mild depression. Lavender also promotes relaxation and improves sleep, making it especially helpful when anxiety is accompanied by insomnia or nighttime restlessness. In addition, it can ease physical symptoms of anxiety, with studies showing that lavender use is associated with lower heart rate, blood pressure, and muscle tension, supporting both mental and physical relaxation. If you don't like the taste of the tea or tincture, you can purchase an over-the-counter supplement called CalmAid. The main ingredient is Silexan, the name for orally administered lavender.

Lemon Balm (Melissa officinalis)

Lemon balm is a versatile and widely loved herb, prized for its calming and cognitive benefits. A member of the mint family, it is a hardy perennial that grows easily and often spreads like a weed throughout your yard! It reseeds itself and spreads by roots, much like mint, making it a low maintenance but vigorous grower.

Traditionally used to soothe the nervous system, ease anxiety and mild depression, and support restful sleep, it has a light, citrusy aroma that pairs beautifully with other herbs. I love sipping a cup of lemon balm and lavender tea before bed; it helps me gently drift off to sleep.

In addition to its calming properties, lemon balm may also support brain health. According to herbalists David Winston and Steven Maimes in their book Adaptogens: "Herbs for Strength, Stamina, and Stress Relief", lemon balm can enhance cognitive function, elevate mood, and ease symptoms of mild to moderate Alzheimer's disease, particularly forgetfulness and irritability.

> **CAUTION:** In large quantities, lemon balm can interfere with thyroid function and thyroid medications, such as Synthroid.

Chamomile (Matricaria recutita)

This gentle and beautiful herb is widely recognized for its calming effects on both the mind and body. It has been traditionally used to ease anxiety, and modern research supports its benefits. It may also help relieve physical symptoms of anxiety, such as tension, restlessness, and sleep disturbances. It is particularly effective for GI-based anxiety and other digestive issues such as irritable bowel syndrome (IBS), acid reflux (GERD), constipation, or diarrhea, all of which can be induced by stress. Due to its gentle nature, it can be given to children. It can be taken as a tea, tincture or capsules.

> **CAUTION:** Avoid chamomile if you have allergies to pollen-bearing plants such as ragweed, chrysanthemums, marigolds, or daisies.

Hops (Humulus lupus)

Hops, commonly known for its role in beer, is also a potent herbal sedative used to support relaxation and sleep. It is a great help when anxiety contributes to restlessness, irritability, or difficulty falling asleep. Hops also works well for those who experience stress in the digestive system, offering relief from gut tension or a nervous stomach. Additionally, it contains mild estrogenic compounds that may help alleviate menstrual or hormone-related symptoms, particularly when these disrupt sleep or mood. Available as a tea, tincture, or capsule, hops is often blended with other calming herbs, such as valerian or passionflower. Due to its strong sedative action, it is best taken in the evening to promote deep, uninterrupted rest.

> **CAUTION:** Due to its sedative properties, it is not recommended during pregnancy, breastfeeding, or alongside other sedative medications without professional guidance.

Kava (Piper methysticum)

Kava is a traditional South Pacific herb celebrated for its powerful calming and anxiety-relieving effects. Extracted from the root of the kava plant, it acts directly on the central nervous system to reduce feelings of fear, panic, and mental restlessness, helping to soothe anxiety without impairing mental clarity or focus. By promoting a deep sense of relaxation and physical ease, kava supports both the mind and body, making it particularly effective for managing acute episodes of anxiety.

It is also commonly used as a gentle bedtime tea to help those who struggle with falling asleep due to nervous tension.

> **CAUTION:** Kava can act as a strong sedative at higher doses, so it should be used in moderation and not taken daily for extended periods without professional supervision. Concerns about liver toxicity are primarily linked to products made from non-root parts of the plant or low-quality extracts. To minimize risk, use only high-quality preparations made from the root and purchased from reputable sources. Avoid kava if you have liver disease or are taking medications that are processed by the liver, unless advised by your healthcare provider.

Fresh Milky Oat (Avena sativa)

This herb has been used for centuries and is highly effective for easing anxiety, particularly when it occurs alongside irritability or nervous exhaustion. It is especially beneficial for those who find themselves easily overwhelmed, where even minor issues can trigger feelings of anxiety and nervousness. It comes from the same plant as oatmeal, oat straw, and rolled oats, but its calming effects are uniquely different. Unlike the common food forms, fresh milky oat specifically targets the nervous system, providing gentle nourishment and support that helps soothe frazzled nerves, reduce tension, and restore a sense of balance and resilience during stressful times.

> **CAUTION:** Do not use fresh milky oat if you have celiac disease or gluten sensitivity.

Passionflower (Passiflora incarnata)

Passionflower is a gentle herb known for its sedative properties and is widely used to help alleviate nervousness, anxiety, and insomnia. By calming the nervous system, it promotes relaxation and supports restful sleep, making it a popular natural remedy for those struggling with stress-related sleep disturbances. In addition to its calming effects on the mind, passionflower also acts as an antispasmodic, helping to soothe and relax the muscles of the digestive tract. This can ease digestive discomfort such as cramping or indigestion that often accompanies anxiety. Because of its sedative nature, passionflower can cause drowsiness, so it is best reserved for use in the evening or before bedtime rather than during the day.

Rose (Rosa damascena)

In the beautiful Indian medical system of Ayurveda, the rose is a cooling flower that is wonderful for the hot summer months. It soothes the heart and helps heal grief, allowing you to move forward and be present. It can help reduce inflammation and associated emotions, such as rage and anger. When dealing with anxiety, we could benefit from some heart healing, and this is just the herb to do it. Rose blends well with chamomile for a lovely tea.

Skullcap (Scutellaria lateriflora)

Like lemon balm, this herb belongs to the mint family and shares many of its soothing qualities. It is especially effective for calming what Buddhists refer to as the "monkey mind," an overactive, restless mind that jumps from one worry to the next, struggling to find peace. By gently quieting this mental chatter, the herb helps promote a sense of calm and mental clarity. It makes a beautiful, fragrant tea to enjoy before bed, supporting relaxation and encouraging a restful night's sleep. While drinking it occasionally can provide immediate soothing effects, the best and most lasting benefits are achieved through consistent daily use, allowing the herb to gradually strengthen the nervous system and improve overall resilience to stress.

Valerian (Valeriana officinalis)

Valerian root is a widely respected herb for calming the nervous system and relieving anxiety, particularly when symptoms include restlessness, muscle tension, or difficulty sleeping. It is especially effective for anxiety linked to physical tension and agitation, and is helpful when anxiety interferes with sleep. Often included in calming herbal blends alongside gentler nervines, such as lemon balm or passionflower, valerian creates a balanced and soothing effect.

> **CAUTION:** Although generally safe, valerian can cause some people to feel excessively sleepy or, in rare cases, more wired instead of calm. Therefore, it's best to use it in small amounts and consult a professional if you plan to take it regularly.

Adaptogens

Adaptogenic herbs are a class of botanicals that help the body adapt to physical, emotional, and environmental stressors in a safe, balanced, and rejuvenating way. When anxiety throws the nervous system off balance, adaptogens gently support the body's return to equilibrium. They enhance vitality, bolster the immune system, and promote long-term resilience. In Ayurveda, these herbs are known as Rasayanas, which translates to "path of essence," a reference to their deeply nourishing and restorative qualities. Similarly, in Traditional Chinese Medicine, tonifying herbs are used for the same purpose, though the terminology and classifications may differ.

Although the term "adrenal fatigue" isn't officially recognized by conventional medicine, it describes a very real pattern of symptoms, including chronic fatigue, mood imbalances, insomnia, muscle aches, poor digestion, cravings for salt and sugar, and brain fog. It's similar to running a car on empty.

Your body's stress response system becomes depleted. Given the relentless pace of modern life, constant connectivity, and limited opportunities to rest, it's no surprise that so many people experience these symptoms.

Adaptogens offer gentle yet powerful support for this kind of burnout. Taken daily, they can help restore hormonal balance, regulate the stress response, and bring the body back to homeostasis, which is the body's natural process of maintaining stable internal conditions, such as temperature, hormones, and energy levels, so that everything functions properly. It's how the body stays balanced, even during stress or change. Depending on the individual, additional herbs can be layered in to address specific challenges such as anxiety, restlessness, insomnia, difficulty focusing, PTSD, or conditions rooted in the gut or thyroid.

Ashwagandha (Withania somnifera)

This Ayurvedic herb from India is widely recognized for its effectiveness in managing anxiety, nervousness, and insomnia. In a study involving sixty-two participants, those taking ashwagandha showed significant improvements in anxiety and stress compared to those given a placebo. Beyond anxiety relief, ashwagandha is also used to address fatigue, cardiovascular issues, skin problems, muscle strength, energy levels, and sexual function in both men and women. As a nervine, it works gradually, so it's best to allow up to four weeks to experience its full benefits.

> **CAUTION:** Avoid ashwagandha if you are allergic to plants in the nightshade family, have hyperthyroidism, or have hemochromatosis (excess iron).

Holy Basil/Tulsi (Ocimum sanctum)

Holy basil, also known as Tulsi, is another highly esteemed herb from India and a relative of the familiar sweet basil. It is renowned for its benefits in managing stress, hypertension, cognitive function, and improving blood flow. Additionally, it supports cardiovascular health, helps lower blood sugar levels, and alleviates respiratory issues like coughs and bronchitis, serving as an expectorant. Holy basil can soothe the mind and combat fatigue and is considered a versatile herb for overall well-being. It also acts as an antidepressant.

Of all the adaptogens available, ashwagandha and holy basil are my go-to recommendations for managing stress and anxiety. While many adaptogenic herbs are effective, these two have consistently shown the most profound and reliable results in my personal experience with clients.

Herbal Teas

Caffeine is well-known for causing jitteriness, and it can be especially problematic for those dealing with anxiety. Beverages like coffee, tea, and soda, particularly the latter due to its high sugar content, can exacerbate anxiety symptoms. Try reducing your daily caffeine intake. A good starting point is to avoid caffeine after 6 p.m. For example, if you usually drink three cups of caffeinated beverages a day, try cutting back to two cups and then gradually decreasing your intake further. You can also substitute with decaf.

Herbal tea is a caffeine-free alternative that allows you to incorporate calming herbs into your daily life. I like Traditional Medicinals, Organic India, Yogi, and Buddha Teas. Additionally, you can experiment with brewing your herbal blends using real tea leaves, incorporating any of the herbs discussed earlier. Get creative by combining one or more herbs tailored to address your specific needs.

There are two methods of preparing herbal tea: infusion and decoction. An infusion is made with the leaves and flowers, which are the delicate parts of the plants. Lavender, lemon balm, rose, Tulsi, and chamomile are examples of herbs that would be infused. A decoction is made with roots, barks, and berries, such as ashwagandha, elderberry, kava, and astragalus.

Making an Infusion

- Bring eight ounces of water to a boil.
- Turn off the heat and add one to two teaspoons of herbs.
- Steep for at least five to seven minutes, but up to twenty if you like strong tea.
- Strain out the herbs.
- Add a little honey, maple syrup, or coconut sugar for added sweetness, if desired.
- Enjoy!

Making a Decoction

- Add two teaspoons of herbs to sixteen ounces of cold water. You can double the recipe to have enough tea to enjoy throughout the day.
- Bring the herbs and water to a low boil.
- Cover the pot and simmer for thirty minutes.
- Remove the decoction from the heat and allow it to cool.
- Strain out the herbs.
- Add a little honey, maple syrup, or coconut sugar for added sweetness, if desired.
- Enjoy!

CAUTION: Consult your doctor before taking any herbal supplements.

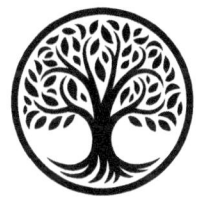

> "The highest ideal of therapy is to restore health rapidly, gently, permanently; to remove and destroy the whole disease in the shortest, surest, least harmful way, according to clearly comprehensive principles."
>
> — SAMUEL HAHNEMANN

CHAPTER 15

Homeopathy

Homeopathy is a system of medicine designed to stimulate the body's natural healing abilities. It was developed over two hundred years ago by German physician Samuel Hahnemann, who became increasingly disillusioned with conventional medicine. He found it not only ineffective at times but, in some cases, harmful. He began to question whether what he had learned in medical school was truly helping people get better. His frustration deepened as he watched patients suffer and sometimes even die from the very treatments meant to cure them. The tragic loss of his son was the final breaking point, prompting him to leave the medical establishment altogether.

In search of a better way, Hahnemann began experimenting with extremely small doses of medicines to see if they could still be effective without causing harmful side effects. This led to what's now known as Hahnemann's Law of the Minimum Dose, the idea that the more diluted a remedy is, the more powerful its healing effect can be. For this reason, homeopathic remedies are given in highly diluted forms.

Homeopathy is also based on the Law of Similars, also known as the concept of "like cures like." This means that a substance which causes symptoms in a healthy person might be used in tiny amounts to help heal those same symptoms in someone who is ill. A modern example of this concept is the flu vaccine, which utilizes a small amount of the flu virus to help the body develop immunity.

One of the key benefits of homeopathic remedies is that they generally do not interfere with other medications and rarely produce side effects. Homeopathy also doesn't just treat a disease label; it looks at the whole person and their unique set of symptoms. It's a holistic approach that considers the mind, body, and spirit, and works with the body's innate healing intelligence.

Hahnemann went on to develop and test more than a hundred remedies. Over the years, homeopathy has garnered the support of many notable figures, including members of the British Royal Family and Mahatma Gandhi, who appreciated its gentle, individualized approach to healing.

A practitioner will begin by analyzing the source of your anxiety to determine the most appropriate remedy. For instance, if your anxiety stems from a specific situation like public speaking, you would receive a different remedy than if it were related to grief from losing a loved one. For generalized anxiety, one helpful remedy is Boiron's Sedalia or StressCalm. Dissolve two tablets under your tongue up to three times a day when feeling restless or anxious.

Homeopathic medicines come in small, white pellets that dissolve under the tongue, although some remedies, such as cough medicine, are available in liquid form or tinctures. They act quickly without causing drowsiness, making them ideal for use at work or to keep in your handbag or pocket. Boiron also offers a stress kit designed for different times of the day to help with stress and anxiety.

Homeopathy is also safe for children and pets. Check the resources at the end of the book to find a practitioner in your area.

CAUTION: While homeopathic remedies are generally considered safe and free of drug interactions, there are a few important cautions to keep in mind. They should not be used as a substitute for seeking medical care, especially in serious or life-threatening conditions. Some over-the-counter products labeled as "homeopathic" may contain herbs or active ingredients that could interact with medications, so always check the label carefully. It's also wise to consult a qualified practitioner to ensure the remedy is appropriate for your unique health needs.

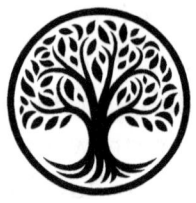

> "Our essential nature is usually overshadowed by the activity of the mind."
>
> — PATANJALI

CHAPTER 16

Meditation

When most people hear the word "meditation," they may envision incense, monks on mountaintops, or individuals sitting cross-legged in silence for hours. And while those images sound wonderful, meditation doesn't have to look or feel that way to be effective. Meditation and mindfulness are practical tools anyone can use to bring more calm, clarity, and presence into everyday life.

First, let's clear up a common misconception. Mindfulness and meditation are closely related but not identical. Mindfulness is simply the act of paying deliberate, non-judgmental attention to the present moment, your thoughts, feelings, body sensations, or surroundings. It can happen anytime, whether you're driving, eating, walking, or washing dishes. Meditation, on the other hand, is a formal practice that helps you build the skill of mindfulness by training your attention, much like exercising your brain.

Meditation includes many styles, from mindfulness meditation, where you focus on your breath or bodily sensations, to loving-kindness (metta) meditation, which cultivates compassion for yourself and others, to Transcendental Meditation (TM), which involves silently repeating a mantra. The key is finding what resonates with you and fits into your life.

If you think, "I can't meditate because my mind won't stop racing," you're not alone. The truth is that a busy mind is exactly why meditation is so helpful. It can be hard to stop the constant stream of thoughts. That's perfectly okay. Thoughts will always come and go. On average, we generate between 60,000 to 80,000 thoughts each day, so stopping them entirely is impossible and impractical. Meditation teaches us to relate to our thoughts differently and to notice them without getting caught up or overwhelmed. It's less about emptying your mind and more about creating space within it.

Have you ever become so absorbed in an activity, whether it be gardening, reading, cooking, or even washing dishes, that you lost track of time? That's a form of meditation. It's about being fully present and engaged, which mindfulness encourages.

In today's fast-paced world, with constant distractions and mental clutter, meditation offers a way to pause, clear the mind, and find balance. Even dedicating five to twenty minutes a day can bring significant benefits, reducing stress and improving emotional well-being. Over time, meditation can help quiet the mental chatter and bring moments of clarity and peace.

Many respected teachers and scientists have helped make mindfulness and meditation both accessible and evidence based. Jon Kabat-Zinn, a pioneer who introduced Mindfulness-Based Stress Reduction (MBSR) to mainstream medicine, defines mindfulness as "paying attention, on purpose, in the present moment, non-judgmentally." Neuroscientists like Judson Brewer study how mindfulness helps break habits and ease anxiety.

Neuroscientist Sam Harris and psychologists like Jack Kornfield, Tara Brach, and Daniel Goleman have helped translate these ancient practices into everyday life.

You don't need to sit perfectly still or carve out hours of silence to practice meditation. Start small, be kind to yourself, and remember that there's no "right" or "wrong" way to do it. Focus on your breath, gently returning your attention when it wanders, and notice the little moments of presence that already occur in your day.

Ultimately, meditation and mindfulness aren't about escaping life. They're about showing up fully for it, cultivating a little more peace and joy right here, in the middle of everything.

Where in your day can you pause and truly pay attention? What might it feel like to meet this very moment with kindness and curiosity?

Here's a simple practice to try:

Next time you're in the shower, ask yourself, are you really here, or are you already planning your day? Notice the feel of the water on your skin, the warmth surrounding you, and your feet grounded against the tub. Just focus on that experience. And when your mind wanders (because it will), gently guide it back. That's the heart of the practice.

Whether you're new to meditation or have been practicing for years, remember this: simply noticing is enough. Every moment is a fresh start. Mindfulness isn't a goal to achieve; it's something we return to again and again, breath by breath, thought by thought, with compassion.

I'll leave you with one final thought from Jon Kabat-Zinn:

"You can't stop the waves, but you can learn to surf."

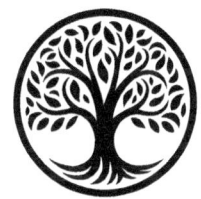

"The power of music to integrate and cure... is quite fundamental. It is the profoundest nonchemical medication."

— Dr. Oliver Sacks

CHAPTER 17

Music Therapy

Who doesn't love music? It's been a part of my life for as long as I can remember. What always amazes me is that while I might forget what I had for lunch yesterday, I can still remember every word of a song I loved decades ago, without missing a beat!

As more people seek integrative ways to support their mental health, music therapy is stepping into the spotlight as a powerful tool for easing anxiety. Music connects with us on such a deep emotional level. With more research confirming its benefits, it's becoming a meaningful complement to traditional therapy.

Much like certain aromas, music has the power to transport us to a memory, a feeling, even a completely different emotional state. A single song can bring joy, calm, nostalgia, or release. That's why one of the simplest ways to shift your mood is to reach for music you love, especially the kind that lifts your spirits or reminds you of a time when you felt happy, grounded, or free.

Music therapy itself is a formal therapeutic approach led by trained, certified professionals. It includes a range of techniques, such as listening to music, playing instruments, singing, writing songs, or using music as a guide for relaxation or breathwork. Sessions are tailored to support each person's emotional, physical, and mental needs.

Even outside of a therapy setting, simply listening to your favorite music or pairing music with deep breathing or mindfulness exercises can help settle the nervous system and ease anxious thoughts. Music has a unique way of bypassing the analytical mind and going straight to the heart, offering comfort and release.

Music has been an integral part of cultures around the world for centuries. Many ancient cultures incorporated music into rituals and ceremonies to heal physical and emotional ailments. Folk music and traditional healing practices were closely intertwined in many indigenous cultures. Shamanic traditions often involved drumming, chanting, and other musical expressions to induce altered states of consciousness and facilitate healing. In ancient China, traditional Chinese medicine practitioners used specific musical scales, known as the Five Tones, as part of their healing practices.

Music played a central role in community gatherings and festivals in ancient cultures, fostering a sense of unity, connection, and well-being. Dancing and singing together were believed to promote harmony and balance within the community. These ancient traditions inspire modern approaches to music therapy and sound healing today.

Dr. Suzanne Hanser, founding chair emerita of Berklee's Music Therapy Department and president of the International Association for Music & Medicine, conducted an experiment demonstrating that people suffering from a combination of severe depression and high anxiety respond more positively when music is included in their treatment. Ten patients were visited at home by a therapist who used music to help them relax their minds and bodies. Ten more were coached by phone to develop their own program. Ten others received no music therapy as part of their treatment and served as comparison subjects.

Dr. Hanser found results that clearly showed that the people being treated for depression and anxiety were helped using music. "The benefit lasted not just for a day or two, but for at least nine months, according to the results of a follow-up study," said Hanser.

Research continues to support music therapy as an effective tool for reducing anxiety. A large meta-analysis of over 70 studies found that music therapy significantly reduced anxiety symptoms across a wide range of mental health conditions (Bradt et al., 2016). Similarly, music interventions have been shown to ease anxiety and boost mood in patients undergoing medical procedures like surgery or chemotherapy (Chan et al., 2018). Even in older adults with dementia, group music therapy helped lower both anxiety and depression levels (Lee et al., 2018).

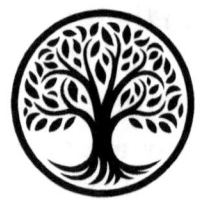

> "There is no need for temples, no need for complicated philosophies. My brain and my heart are my temples; my philosophy is kindness."
>
> — H.H. THE DALAI LAMA

CHAPTER 18

Religion and Spirituality

According to *Spirituality for Dummies* by Sharon Janis, "Spirituality is the wellspring of divinity that pulsates, dances, and flows as the source and essence of every soul. Spirituality relates more to your personal search, to finding greater meaning and purpose in your existence. Religion is most often used to describe an organized group or culture that has generally been sparked by the fire of a spiritual or divine soul. Religions usually aim to present specific teachings and doctrines while nurturing and propagating a particular way of life."

While they complement each other beautifully, spirituality and therapy are not the same, and that's a good thing. Each offers something unique, and together, they can be especially powerful in easing anxiety.

Managing anxiety often requires more than surface-level fixes. It asks us to look inward, to explore what's really going on beneath the stress and overwhelm. That's where spirituality can play a deeply meaningful role.

The Buddha taught that both our suffering and our happiness begin in the mind. In other words, when we shift how we see and respond to our inner world, we can change our experience of life itself. Spirituality encourages this kind of self-reflection. It nudges us to pause, to become curious about our thoughts and patterns, and to grow from what we discover.

When anxiety shows up, instead of pushing it away, we can learn to ask: What's behind this? What needs attention? That gentle curiosity, paired with self-compassion, not only helps soothe anxiety but also helps us live more connected, grounded, and meaningful lives.

In his book *"Earth's Elders: The Wisdom of the World's Oldest People"*, Jerry Friedman interviewed individuals who were over 110 years old, known as supercentenarians. One powerful theme that emerged was a deep sense of spirituality. While their beliefs and practices varied, nearly all of them shared a strong spiritual connection. For many, spirituality offered a sense of purpose and meaning, as well as a connection to something greater, whether they referred to it as God, a higher power, or simply the mystery of life itself.

Dan Buettner, Founder of The Blue Zones, National Geographic Fellow, and #1 *New York Times* Bestselling Author, discovered places around the world where people live the longest. He shares his research in a series of books on the Blue Zones, and a four-part Netflix series titled "Live to 100: Secrets of the Blue Zones."

He states that "People who pay attention to their spiritual side have lower rates of cardiovascular disease, depression, stress, and suicide, and their immune systems seem to work better. To a certain extent, adherence to a religion allows them to relinquish the stresses of everyday life to a higher power."

Both religion and spirituality offer a perspective that transcends daily challenges, the stresses, obligations, bills, and work that often contribute to feelings of anxiety or depression. While religion and spirituality alone don't eradicate mental health issues, they serve as valuable tools for coping.

These practices encourage introspection and inspire a commitment to helping others during challenging times. Engaging in charitable activities and volunteer work has been shown to boost levels of endorphins, often referred to as "feel-good hormones," which can help alleviate anxiety and stress. Finding deeper meaning in life and cultivating gratitude nurtures a sense of contentment and greater inner peace.

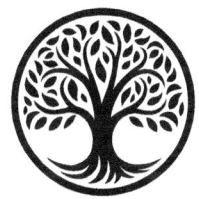

> "Innocent sleep. Sleep that soothes away all our worries. Sleep that puts each day to rest. Sleep that relieves the weary laborer and heals hurt minds."
>
> — WILLIAM SHAKESPEARE

CHAPTER 19

Sleep

In an initial consultation, I ask my clients, "How is your sleep?" Surprisingly, over 95% typically respond with either "Not great," "Terrible," or "I don't sleep." Stress and an overactive mind are the most common reasons they give when I ask why.

Sleep is essential for both our physical health and mental well-being, yet many of us underestimate just how much it affects anxiety. Research shows a strong connection between poor sleep and increased anxiety symptoms. Up to 90% of people with anxiety disorders struggle with getting enough restful sleep.

For example, a study in the *Journal of Sleep Research* found that people with generalized anxiety disorder have a harder time falling asleep compared to those without anxiety. This difficulty often feeds back into their anxiety, creating a frustrating cycle.

Another study published in the Journal of Clinical Sleep Medicine showed that people with insomnia are more likely to develop anxiety and depression than those who sleep well.

Why does this happen? Sleep is crucial for managing our emotions. Without enough sleep, our ability to regulate emotions becomes impaired. Specifically, lack of sleep can over-activate the amygdala, the part of the brain responsible for processing emotions, making us more reactive to stress. Plus, sleep deprivation raises cortisol, the body's stress hormone, making anxiety feel even worse.

Getting good sleep isn't just about feeling rested; it's a vital part of calming the mind and keeping anxiety in check.

In my work with clients facing sleep challenges, I often recommend applying the solutions outlined in this book. Chapter sixteen discusses the powerful impact of meditation. For those new to it, I suggest starting with just five minutes daily, gradually increasing to twenty minutes twice daily over time. Keeping a television, computer, or phone in the bedroom can worsen the problem, as these devices tend to overstimulate, making it difficult to relax the mind and body. Consistency in daily routines is crucial for achieving quality sleep.

Changing your routines and habits can feel overwhelming. If you're looking for guidance, working with a health and wellness coach might be just the support you need. We're here to help you build strategies, stay motivated, and hold you accountable as you set and reach your goals, creating lasting, positive change. Remember, everyone needs a little help sometimes, and support is always within reach.

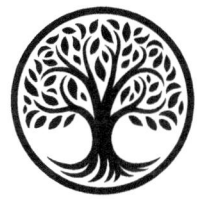

> "Social connections are the greatest predictor of happiness, even more than money or status."
>
> — Robert Waldinger

CHAPTER 20

Social Connection

Who doesn't feel better after a good chat with a friend or a fun evening out with loved ones? We often think self-care is all about eating right, exercising, and getting enough sleep, but social connection is just as essential. One landmark study found that lacking social ties poses a bigger risk to our health than obesity, smoking, or high blood pressure. Having a strong support network not only helps reduce anxiety but also boosts your immune system, speeds up recovery from illness, and can increase your chances of living longer by up to 50%!

People with strong social connections tend to handle stress more effectively, thanks to the many ways support from others helps us cope:

- **Emotional Support:** Being part of a caring community offers comfort and reassurance during tough times. Knowing you're not alone can ease feelings of anxiety and stress.

- **Sense of Belonging:** Feeling connected to others fosters a sense of belonging, which can help reduce loneliness and isolation, two major contributors to anxiety.
- **Shared Experiences:** When you share your struggles with people who truly understand, it validates your feelings and lessens anxiety. Support groups, for example, provide safe spaces to open up and find community.
- **Encouragement and Motivation:** Friends and communities often inspire us to keep going, encouraging healthy habits and positive coping strategies.
- **Resource Sharing:** Strong social networks also provide access to valuable resources, such as information about mental health, coping tools, and relaxation techniques.

Dr. Vivek Murthy, the former U.S. Surgeon General, has highlighted the profound impact of loneliness and anxiety on public health. In his book *"Together: The Healing Power of Human Connection in a Sometimes Lonely World"*, Dr. Murthy discusses how loneliness can exacerbate anxiety and other mental health issues. He emphasizes the importance of building strong social connections to combat these feelings. According to Dr. Murthy, fostering community and meaningful relationships is essential for improving mental health and overall well-being. He advocates for societal efforts to reduce stigma and promote mental health support networks.

There are many ways to foster community, whether by joining a support group, staying connected to friends and family (those who don't stress you out!), or engaging in community activities to build new connections.

Peer support groups and group coaching have shown positive results. These groups provide a platform for individuals to share their experiences and coping strategies, reducing feelings of isolation.

Online communities have become a vital source of support for those with anxiety. These virtual platforms offer anonymity and accessibility, making it easier to seek help and connect with others who face similar challenges. A study by Naslund et al. (2016) found that participation in online mental health communities led to increased social support and a reduction in feelings of isolation among users. Online forums, social media groups, and mental health apps provide various forms of support, including emotional encouragement, informational resources, and peer interactions. These communities were lifesavers during COVID.

The bottom line is sometimes it takes a village, and we all need help and support from time to time, so why not ask for it?

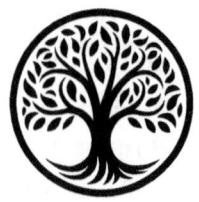

> "Acceptance doesn't mean resignation; it means understanding that something is what it is and that there's got to be a way through it."
>
> — Michael J. Fox

CHAPTER 21

Acceptance and Commitment Therapy (ACT)

Acceptance and Commitment Therapy (ACT), developed by psychologist Steven C. Hayes in the 1980s, offers a fresh and empowering way to understand and work with anxiety. Rooted in contextual behavioral science, ACT shifts the focus from trying to get rid of uncomfortable thoughts and feelings to learning how to relate to them differently.

Rather than fighting against anxiety, an approach that can often make it worse, ACT teaches us to accept our internal experiences (like anxious thoughts, emotions, and bodily sensations) without judgment. Traditional therapies usually emphasize controlling or reducing symptoms, such as using cognitive restructuring to challenge negative thoughts or exposure therapy to desensitize fear responses. While these can be helpful, ACT proposes a different goal: psychological flexibility.

Psychological flexibility means being able to stay present with whatever shows up internally, such as anxiety, and still take meaningful action in alignment with your values. In this model, the goal isn't to eliminate anxiety but to change the way you respond to it.

ACT recognizes that struggling to avoid or suppress anxiety can intensify it. The more we resist or try to escape it, the more power it seems to hold over us. Instead, ACT invites us to accept anxiety's presence and view it as a signal, not a stop sign—guiding us to pay attention to what matters most.

By learning to accept anxiety and take committed action anyway, you begin to reclaim your life from fear's grip. This approach fosters a healthier, more compassionate, and more adaptive relationship with anxiety, one rooted in growth, resilience, and authenticity.

ACT is Based on Six Core Processes:

1. **Acceptance**

    Acceptance means noticing and allowing your full range of thoughts, feelings, and sensations without trying to avoid, change, or control them. In ACT, this involves letting anxiety be present without judgment or resistance. For instance, if you notice your heart racing before a big presentation, instead of fighting that feeling or telling yourself "I shouldn't be nervous," you simply acknowledge it: "I'm feeling anxious right now." Often, trying to fight or control anxiety only makes it worse. By accepting anxiety instead of labeling it as "bad" or "unacceptable," you reduce its power over you. Acceptance doesn't mean that anxiety feels comfortable; it means you allow it to be there while still choosing to live life. It's about making space for your emotions without trying to resist, avoid, or change them.

2. **Cognitive Defusion**

   This technique helps you step back from distressing thoughts and change how you relate to them, which makes them less impactful. Imagine you have the thought, "I'm going to fail this test." Instead of believing it as an absolute truth, you might say, "I'm having the thought that I'm going to fail." By putting some distance between you and the thought, it loses its grip. Another example: when a negative thought pops up, try singing it to a silly tune or saying it in a cartoon voice. This can help you see the thought as just words, not facts, which lowers its emotional impact.

3. **Present Moment Awareness**

   Also known as mindfulness, this means fully engaging with what is happening right now, without judgment or trying to change it. Picture yourself eating a meal: instead of rushing or scrolling on your phone, you focus on the taste, texture, and smell of the food. This simple act grounds you in the moment. Mindfulness helps you avoid getting overwhelmed by worries about the future or regrets about the past. When anxiety strikes, try focusing on your breath or noticing the sensations in your body. These small practices calm your mind and let you observe anxiety without getting lost in it.

4. **Self-as-Context**

   This concept teaches that you are not your thoughts, feelings, or experiences. Rather than identifying with them, like thinking, "I am anxious," self-as-context invites you to step back and observe. You might instead say, "I'm noticing the feeling of anxiety again." This subtle shift helps you recognize that your emotions and thoughts come and go, like clouds passing through the sky. Seeing yourself as the observer of your thoughts and feelings gives you space to respond with more calm and clarity, rather than reacting based on fear, stress, or habit.

5. **Values Clarification**

    When anxiety strikes, it's easy to lose sight of what really matters to us. Values clarification is about reconnecting with your core beliefs and what gives your life meaning. Say you deeply value friendship but feel nervous about reaching out. Instead of avoiding social situations, consider sending a text to a friend or attending a small gathering. Even though anxiety is still there, acting according to your values helps you build purpose and shows that anxiety doesn't define you.

6. **Committed Action**

    Committed action means taking small, meaningful steps toward your values and goals, even when anxiety is loud in your head. It's not about waiting until the fear goes away but choosing to move forward with it. For example, if anxiety tells you, "You'll embarrass yourself at the gym," committed action might be lacing up your sneakers and walking around the block instead. It could be joining a friend for a short yoga video at home. The step doesn't have to be big. What matters is that it's in the direction of what's important to you. Taking action, even while feeling anxious, builds confidence over time. It's how you show yourself: "Anxiety is here, but it doesn't get to make all the decisions."

ACT doesn't promise to erase anxiety. What it offers is a new way to move with it, with more grace, clarity, and confidence in who you are.

Look for a licensed therapist, counselor, social worker, or mental health professional with training and experience in ACT. Although there is no official certification for ACT, many practitioners gain expertise through workshops, peer counseling, and specialized training. Take the time to talk with potential practitioners to make sure you feel comfortable and confident in their care.

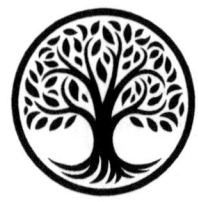

> "Give a man a fish and you feed him for a day. Teach him how to fish and you feed him for a lifetime."
>
> — Lao Tzu

CHAPTER 22

Biofeedback

In the 1960s and 1970s, something fascinating caught the attention of scientists. They started studying monks and yogis who had spent years practicing deep meditation. What they found was nothing short of remarkable. Simply by using their minds, they could slow their breathing, lower their heart rate, and even adjust their body temperature. They had figured out how to shift the body's automatic stress response into a state of deep calm.

Biofeedback was born. Think of it as a way to get a behind-the-scenes look at what's going on in your body, things like muscle tension, heart rate, and breathing, especially when you're under stress. With the help of small sensors and a screen showing your body's reactions in real time, you start to notice patterns that were always there but often ignored. Maybe your shoulders tense every time your phone buzzes, or your breath gets shallow when you're overwhelmed. Once you see it, you can change it. That's the power of awareness.

Biofeedback is like having a coach for your nervous system. It helps you recognize when your body is going into fight-or-flight mode and teaches you how to guide yourself back to a more balanced and calm state. Instead of being swept away by anxiety, you learn how to work with it using real, accessible tools.

Anxiety doesn't just live in your thoughts, it shows up in your body, too. A pounding heart, tight muscles, sweaty palms, and shallow breathing are your body's way of sounding the alarm, even when there's no real danger. But when these alarms go off too often or without warning, they can feel overwhelming. That's where biofeedback really shines.

One key focus of biofeedback is heart rate variability (HRV), the slight, natural variation in the time between each heartbeat. A flexible, resilient nervous system has higher HRV, meaning your body can shift easily between calm and stress. When HRV is low, it's often a sign that stress is in the driver's seat. The good news? You can train your body to increase HRV through simple techniques like slow, steady breathing and mindful awareness. With practice, you start to feel more grounded and centered, even when life throws curveballs your way.

Biofeedback can also track muscle tension through a technique called electromyography (EMG). If you've ever noticed your shoulders creeping up to your ears when you're anxious, that's muscle tension at work. Seeing it in real time helps you learn how to release it. Another tool, electrodermal activity, measures sweat gland activity, which increases when you're stressed. Tracking your breathing patterns can also reveal when they've become shallow or erratic so that you can shift back to deeper, more calming breaths.

Sessions often include tools such as slow breathing, progressive muscle relaxation, mindfulness, and visualization. These aren't just fluffy self-care ideas; they're powerful ways to signal to your body that it's safe. With practice, these skills begin to show up in daily life. You might catch yourself breathing differently in traffic or relaxing your jaw during a tense conversation. Those small shifts add up.

Biofeedback can be used as a standalone treatment or combined with therapy, medication, or lifestyle changes. What's unique about it is that it helps you build awareness and confidence in your ability to calm your body and mind. You don't have to wait for anxiety to spiral. You can learn to step in early, recognize the signs, and gently guide yourself back to center.

That's not just healing, that's empowerment.

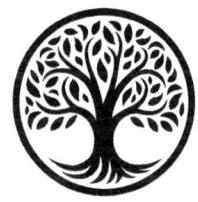

> "If you don't like something, change it. If you can't change it, change your attitude."
>
> — Maya Angelou

CHAPTER 23

Cognitive Behavioral Therapy

If you've ever felt like your thoughts have a mind of their own, racing ahead to the worst-case scenario or spiraling over something small, you're not alone. That's exactly where Cognitive Behavioral Therapy, or CBT, comes in. It's one of the most effective and well-researched tools we have for treating anxiety, and with good reason. It helps you understand how your thoughts, feelings, and behaviors are interconnected and how changing one can impact the others.

Rather than diving into your past or endlessly analyzing your childhood (though that has value in other therapies), CBT is all about what's happening now, what you're thinking in this moment that might be feeding your anxiety. It helps you become more aware of your internal dialogue and the automatic thoughts you barely notice, but that have a significant impact on how you feel. The ones that whisper things like "What if something goes wrong?" or "I can't handle this."

In CBT, you work alongside a therapist to identify those thought patterns and examine them with curiosity, rather than judgment. You're invited to gently challenge your assumptions and ask, "Is this actually true?" You begin to untangle the knots of worry and create space for more balanced thinking, thoughts that still acknowledge your concerns but aren't ruled by fear.

Here's the beauty of it: when you start thinking differently, you begin to feel different. That's not just an idea; it's something we can measure. Studies show CBT leads to meaningful and lasting changes, not just in mood, but in how the brain processes stress. People often find they don't need to rely as heavily on medication or avoid things that used to cause panic. They feel more capable, more equipped.

One of the more active parts of CBT, especially for phobias or persistent fears, is something called exposure therapy. It means facing what you've been avoiding slowly and intentionally, not all at once, and not without support. The idea isn't to flood yourself with fear, but to prove to your nervous system that you're safe, even when it doesn't feel that way at first. For someone afraid of flying (like me), that might begin with simply watching planes take off, then stepping onto one while it's on the ground, and eventually taking a short flight. Step by step, your brain learns there's less to fear than it once believed.

CBT also provides you with practical tools that you can carry with you, such as calming breathwork, mindfulness, and relaxation techniques to help regulate your nervous system in real-time. The more you use them, the more natural they become. You might find yourself pausing to breathe during a stressful meeting or shifting your self-talk when panic starts to rise. These moments of awareness become small wins that build your confidence over time.

Most importantly, CBT puts the power back in your hands. It doesn't promise to eliminate anxiety completely, but it does teach you how to navigate it with more ease and clarity. And that shift from feeling powerless to feeling prepared is one of the most healing parts of the journey.

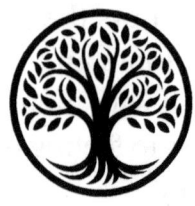

> "The wound is the place the light enters you."
> — RUMI

CHAPTER 24

Eye Movement Desensitization and Reprocessing (EMDR)

Eye Movement Desensitization and Reprocessing (EMDR) is a psychotherapy approach designed to help process and heal from traumatic or distressing experiences. Developed in the late 1980s by American psychologist Dr. Francine Shapiro, EMDR involves recalling emotionally charged memories while simultaneously engaging in bilateral stimulation, usually through guided side-to-side eye movements. This process is believed to help the brain reprocess those memories, reducing their emotional intensity and helping them feel less overwhelming.

Dr. Shapiro first noticed the potential of this technique when she observed that her own troubling thoughts seemed to lose their emotional grip after her eyes moved rapidly back and forth. Curious about the effect, she began researching and ultimately developed EMDR into a structured, evidence-based therapeutic method.

EMDR was originally created to treat post-traumatic stress disorder (PTSD), but its use has since expanded to include conditions like anxiety, depression, and phobias, particularly when these issues stem from unresolved past experiences. For anxiety rooted in specific memories or events, EMDR can help reframe those experiences, allowing the nervous system to return to a more regulated and present state. Rather than reliving emotional pain, individuals begin to respond to those memories with greater distance and less distress.

EMDR therapy follows a structured eight-phase process, each phase building on the last to support healing and integration. This structure is part of what makes the therapy so effective. It offers both a roadmap and flexibility tailored to the individual's experience.

History-Taking and Treatment Planning

The journey begins with a thorough examination of the client's background. The therapist gathers information about the person's history, significant life events, symptoms, and emotional challenges. From there, specific memories and themes are identified that will become the focus of the work. This is a collaborative stage, where trust is built and treatment goals are outlined.

Preparation

Before any processing begins, the therapist explains how EMDR works and ensures that the client feels informed and ready to move forward. At this stage, it's also essential to develop tools for emotional regulation. Techniques such as grounding exercises, guided imagery, and breathwork are introduced to help the client stay calm and centered both during and between sessions.

Assessment

Once readiness is established, the therapist and client choose memories to work on. These memories are explored in more detail, including what the client saw, heard, felt, and believed at the time. The client also rates the level of distress connected to the memory and identifies any core negative beliefs it may have created, such as "I'm not safe" or "I'm powerless."

Desensitization

This is where the processing begins. The client recalls the distressing memory while following bilateral stimulation, often in the form of side-to-side eye movements directed by the therapist. As the brain begins to reprocess the event, the emotional intensity starts to decrease. New insights may emerge, and the once-overwhelming memory becomes more tolerable, sometimes surprisingly so.

Installation

Once the distress has lessened, the focus shifts to reinforcing a positive belief to replace the old negative one. For example, "I'm powerless" might be replaced with "I did the best I could" or "I'm in control now." This new belief is repeated and strengthened while the client continues with bilateral stimulation, allowing it to take root at a deeper level.

Body Scan

After installing the positive belief, the client is guided to check in with their body, scanning from head to toe, to notice any leftover physical tension or discomfort. If something surfaces, it may signal that a part of the memory still needs attention, and the therapist will help the client process those sensations until they ease.

Closure

Every session ends with a grounding process to ensure the client leaves feeling safe and stable. The therapist checks in both emotionally and physically, reinforces coping skills, and provides tools to help manage any lingering distress that may surface between sessions. Even if a memory isn't fully processed in one session, the client is supported and prepared for the next step.

Reevaluation

At the start of the next session, the therapist and client review what was previously worked on. Is the memory still emotionally neutral? Does the new belief still feel true? If so, they move on to another target. If not, further work may be done. This phase also enables the therapist to monitor progress and adjust the treatment plan as necessary.

EMDR should always be conducted by a trained and licensed mental health professional. While it's a powerful tool for healing, it requires specialized training to ensure it's used safely and effectively.

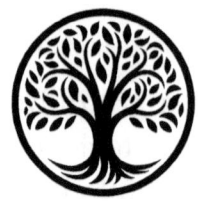

> "When the student is ready, the teacher will appear."
>
> — AUTHOR DEBATED

CHAPTER 25

Health Coaching

Health and well-being coaching is rapidly gaining recognition, and for good reason: it works! Unlike approaches that focus solely on physical health, coaching takes a holistic view of the whole person. It considers your values, goals, work life, physical and mental health, environment, sense of fulfillment, and even your deeper life purpose. This comprehensive perspective enables coaching to address anxiety and other challenges by helping you identify the root causes across all areas of your life. Through ongoing support, accountability, and a safe, nonjudgmental space to explore your concerns, coaching empowers lasting change. You are the CEO of your own life, with the power to make meaningful changes.

Many of us have experienced or know someone who has faced a major life transition, whether related to health, relationships, or career, and struggled to make or sustain meaningful changes. I've worked with people managing chronic conditions like diabetes or recovering from heart attacks, who, despite their strong desire to improve, found it difficult to follow through on the lifestyle shifts their doctors recommended. This is a common experience. Change is hard, and everyone, at some point, needs guidance and encouragement, whether it's to manage anxiety more effectively, increase physical activity, cope with illness, lose weight, improve sleep, transition into a new career, or simplify their living space.

With rising rates of anxiety, depression, and burnout, new approaches to health and wellness are urgently needed. Coaching offers a personalized path for individuals to clarify what they want, set meaningful goals, and take consistent action to improve their quality of life. Through reflective exploration, emotional support, accountability, and practical strategies, clients build momentum and confidence as they move toward their envisioned future.

Healthcare providers often face time constraints that limit their ability to address every aspect of a patient's health or support the behavior changes necessary for lasting progress. Health and well-being coaches serve as essential partners in the care team, allowing doctors to focus on diagnosis and medical treatment while coaches provide the continuous motivation and guidance patients need outside the clinic. When a client is ready to make changes but unsure how to begin, the coach fills that vital role of facilitator and motivator.

The coaching journey begins with an initial session designed to build a strong foundation. This meeting provides an opportunity to establish trust, clarify your support needs, and co-create a tailored plan for your coaching experience. Your coach will introduce the tools and techniques they bring to the process, while helping you gain a deep understanding of who you are, what matters most to you, and what you hope to achieve in your health and well-being.

Benefits of Health Coaching Include:

- **Collaboration** with the client to establish realistic and achievable goals.
- **Awareness Building** to help clients recognize and manage their anxiety more effectively.
- **Regular Check-ins** to provide ongoing emotional support and help clients stay on track with their goals.
- **Accountability Partner** to support clients in sticking to their wellness plans and making necessary adjustments.
- **Safe Space** to provide a non-judgmental, supportive environment for clients to express their feelings and concerns.
- **Empowerment** for clients to actively participate in their mental health journey, building confidence and resilience.
- **Progress Monitoring** for clients to track progress toward goals and adjust as needed for continuous improvement.
- **Feedback Loop** to discuss what's working and what's not, allowing for personalized tweaks to the wellness plan.

By offering a comprehensive, individualized approach, a health and wellness coach can significantly aid in managing anxiety and mental illness, helping clients lead healthier, more balanced lives.

Coaching is not about the coach giving you the answers.

It helps you make changes that you may not otherwise have been able to achieve on your own. The coach asks thought-provoking questions that empower the client to have their own "a-ha" moments, tap into their motivation, take ownership, and start thinking about replacing bad habits and thoughts with good ones. This approach is far more impactful than simply telling someone what to do, as no one likes being told what to do, and it has been proven not to be a good strategy for long-term success.

Contact me for a free discovery call to discuss:

https://www.theholisticroot.com/contact

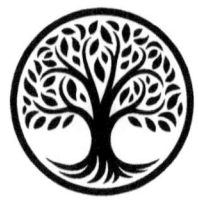

> **"The only person you are destined to become is the person you decide to be."**
>
> — Ralph Waldo Emerson

CHAPTER 26

Therapy

Having support during tough times isn't just helpful. It can be life changing. Sure, friends and family often mean well and can offer comfort, but sometimes what we really need is someone who's not in the middle of our story. Someone who won't judge, who's trained to listen deeply, and who can guide us forward with clarity and compassion. That's where professional support, like therapy, comes in, and it can make all the difference.

Even though conversations about mental health are becoming more common, there's still this lingering stigma, this quiet voice that says, "You should be able to handle this on your own." If you were dealing with a heart condition or diabetes, you wouldn't think twice about getting medical help. So why treat anxiety, depression, or emotional distress any differently?

Getting help isn't weakness. It's wisdom. It's strength. And it's a choice that could change the direction of your healing journey.

When I finally opened up about my own struggle with anxiety, I was amazed by how many people said, "Me too." Some were in the thick of it, while others had been through it and come out the other side, but almost everyone had a story. The thing about anxiety is that it can build up slowly, layer by layer, until one day it just crashes down. You might feel like you're functioning fine, holding it all together, until suddenly you're not, and you can't quite figure out why. That's because anxiety doesn't always have one clear cause. It often stems from a mix of stress, old wounds, daily pressures, and things we don't even realize are weighing us down.

Sometimes, anxiety doesn't travel alone. Depression often tags along, sometimes quietly, sometimes loudly. For me, anxiety eventually gave way to a short bout of depression. And while it was hard, it also helped me understand just how deeply intertwined our emotional struggles can be.

That's why therapy can be so powerful. It's not about being fixed. It's about being seen, heard, and supported. Therapy gives you a private, judgment-free space to say the things you can't always say out loud. A skilled therapist helps you spot the thought patterns that keep you stuck, gently challenges the fears you've come to believe in as truth, and walks alongside you as you start to see yourself and your story in a new light.

More than that, therapy helps you dig beneath the surface. It helps you uncover what's really fueling your anxiety. Old beliefs, hidden fears, unresolved pain and as that insight grows, so does your capacity for change. You don't just cope better. You begin to transform.

Let's not overlook another important benefit therapy offers, which is connection, because anxiety can be isolating. It makes you feel like no one else quite gets it. But in that quiet, supportive space with a therapist, the loneliness begins to lift. You remember that healing doesn't have to be done alone.

No two paths are the same, and a good therapist will tailor their approach to fit you, your past, your relationships, and your pace. Maybe it means revisiting old wounds. Maybe it's about learning how to set boundaries, speak kindly to yourself, or manage the stress that's built up over time. But whatever it is, therapy becomes a space where growth happens.

Over time, you'll likely notice something subtle but powerful. You start responding to life differently. You begin facing challenges with more clarity, calm, and most importantly, with a renewed sense of hope.

Therapy can also complement other treatments, such as medication or lifestyle adjustments, creating a well-rounded approach to anxiety management. When searching for a therapist, it's essential to find someone with whom you feel comfortable, which may involve trying a few options. Ask your doctor or trusted friends for a recommendation.

The website **www.psychologytoday.com** allows you to search for therapists based on your specific needs and insurance.

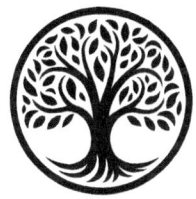

> "Happiness is not something ready-made; it comes from your own actions."
>
> — H.H. the Dalai Lama

CHAPTER 27

What's Next?

Anxiety can surface at any point in life. Sometimes there's a clear reason, and sometimes it sneaks up on you without explanation. But remember that while uncomfortable, anxiety often holds a hidden invitation. It asks us to pause, reflect, and reevaluate how we're living. That's the silver lining. It can wake us up, nudging us toward change, toward healing, and toward living in a way that feels more aligned with who we really are.

The first step is awareness. Begin by taking an honest look at how you spend your time and what you feed your mind. Our modern world floods us with worst-case scenarios, bad news on a loop, outrage in every scroll, and stress disguised as staying "informed." But this constant barrage takes a toll. What you expose yourself to, especially right before bed, can stick with you throughout the night, quietly shaping your thoughts and emotions.

So, start there. Shut off the news. Power down the screens. Instead, fill your space with music that soothes you, words that inspire you, and people who lift you up. You deserve calm, connection, and comfort, and you can create an environment that gives you exactly that.

Next, make space for joy. Reconnect with things that once made you lose track of time. What lit you up as a kid? Was it dancing, painting, singing, cooking, being outside, collecting rocks, or building things with your hands? Whatever it was, do more of that now. Try something new just for fun, take that French class, sign up for pottery, experiment in the kitchen, or even color in a notebook. It doesn't have to be perfect or productive. It just has to make you feel alive again.

When anxiety creeps in, try redirecting your energy. Move your body, play your favorite music, clean out a closet, go for a walk. Action doesn't erase anxiety, but it can shift your energy and give your mind a break.

Also, remember that emotions, especially the difficult ones, can build up like toxins. If you don't let them out, they can get stuck, making your body feel heavy and your spirit even heavier. Letting go of what weighs you down, even slowly and imperfectly, can open up space for healing.

Now is the time to be honest with yourself. What needs to change? What patterns aren't serving you anymore? Not in a judgmental way, but with gentle curiosity. Growth starts with awareness, but it flourishes with kindness, especially toward yourself.

Here are a few simple, powerful ways to shift forward:

- Cultivate a daily practice of gratitude. Take a moment to express, either aloud or to yourself, the aspects of your life that bring you appreciation, your family, friends, pets, good health, home, or anything that brings joy. We all have something to be grateful for.

- Focus on the positive! Shifting to positive thoughts daily can alter your thinking patterns and, in turn, influence your emotions. Be vigilant and catch yourself when negative thoughts arise. Recognize that thoughts and emotions are intricately linked to your physical well-being.
- Engage in acts of service for others. Anxiety often stems from excessive self-focus. Counteract this by redirecting your attention outward. Volunteer or assist those in need. Acts of kindness provide a natural sense of fulfillment and gratitude for your own life.
- If you don't like your life, change it.
- Cultivate a "who cares what anyone thinks of me" attitude.
- Practice forgiveness and kindness.
- Reach out to a good friend or family member when you're feeling anxious. It will make you feel better.
- Try not to judge anyone and treat everyone, including yourself, with compassion.
- Don't hold grudges, and if you do, work to get rid of them.
- Cherish the ones you love.
- Nourish healthy relationships and stay away from toxic ones. Studies show that having a community of friends and family with whom you enjoy spending time is vital to your overall health and longevity.
- Value people, not stuff.
- Get a good night's sleep.
- Commune with nature.
- Listen to some great music and dance.
- Pick your battles.
- Laugh, laugh, laugh!
- Love, love, love!

Anxiety doesn't have to define you.

In fact, it might be the very thing that leads you

back to yourself. Wherever you are right now,

know that you are not alone,

and your path forward is already unfolding,

step by step,

moment by moment.

You've got this!

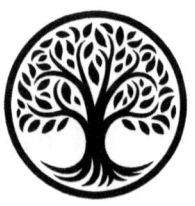

References

Arch, J. J., & Craske, M. G. (2008). Acceptance and Commitment Therapy and Cognitive Behavioral Therapy for Anxiety Disorders: Different Techniques, Similar Mechanisms? *Journal of Consulting and Clinical Psychology*, 76(5), 835-845.

Akhondzadeh, S., Naghavi, H. R., & Vazirian, M. (2001). Passionflower in the treatment of generalized anxiety: A pilot double-blind randomized controlled trial with oxazepam. *Journal of Clinical Pharmaceutical Therapy*, 26, 363-367.

Alternative Medicine Naturopathy. Bach Flower Remedies Case Study - Klinda Weber

American Psychological Association. (2017). *Stress in America: The State of Our Nation.* https://www.apa.org/news/press/releases/stress/2017/state-nation.pdf

Anxiety Disorders Association of America. https://www.adaa.org

Bach Original Flower Remedies. https://www.bachremedies.co.uk/?lang=us

Baglioni, C., Battagliese, G., Feige, B., et al. (2011). Insomnia as a predictor of depression: A meta-analytic evaluation of longitudinal epidemiological studies. *Journal of Affective Disorders*, 135(1-3), 10-19. https://doi.org/10.1016/j.jad.2011.01.011

Balch, Phyllis A. (2000). *Prescription for Nutritional Healing* (Third Edition). Avery.

Bandelow, B., Michaelis, S., & Wedekind, D. (2017). Treatment of Anxiety Disorders. *Dialogues in Clinical Neuroscience*, 19(2), 93–107.

Bazrafshan, M. R., Jokar, M., Shokrpour, N., & Delam, H. (2020). The effect of lavender herbal tea on the anxiety and depression of the elderly: A randomized clinical trial. *Complementary Therapies in Medicine, 50*, 102393. https://doi.org/10.1016/j.ctim.2020.102393

Barati, F., Nasiri, A., Akbari, N., & Sharifzadeh, G. (2016). The Effect of Aromatherapy on Anxiety in Patients. *Nephro-Urology Monthly, 8*(5). https://www.ncbi.nlm.nih.gov/pmc/articles/PMC5111093/

Begeny, C., et al. (2023). *Limiting Social Media Use Decreases Symptoms of Depression and Anxiety.* **Simply Psychology.** Retrieved from https://www.simplypsychology.org/limiting-social-media-use-decreases-depression-anxiety.html

Borkovec, T. D., Shadick, R., & Hopkins, M. (1991). The nature of normal and pathological worry. In R. M. Rapee & D. H. Barlow (Eds.), *Chronic anxiety, generalized anxiety disorder, and mixed anxiety depression* (pp. 29-51). New York: Guilford Press.

Borkovec, T. D., Whisman, M. A., & Durham, T. (1994). Cognitive behavioral therapy treatment for generalized anxiety disorder. Research conducted at Pennsylvania State University.

Bradt, J., Dileo, C., Magill, L., & Teague, A. (2016). Music interventions for improving psychological and physical outcomes in cancer patients. *Cochrane Database of Systematic Reviews, (8)*, CD006911. https://doi.org/10.1002/14651858.CD006911.pub3

Brennan, D. (2020). How Music Affects Mental Health. *WebMD.* https://www.webmd.com/mental-health/how-music-affects-mental-health

Brown, R. P., & Gerbarg, P. L. (2000). Integrative psychopharmacology: A practical approach to herbs and nutrients in psychiatry. In P. R. Muskin (Ed.), *Complementary and alternative medicine and psychiatry (Review of Psychiatry Series, 19)*(1), 1-66. Washington: American Psychiatric Press.

Buchbauer, G., Jirovetz, L., & Jager, W. (1993). Fragrance compounds and essential oils with sedative effects upon inhalation. *Journal of Pharmaceutical Science, 88*(6), 660-664. Retrieved abstract from PUBMED.

Budd, K. (2019, September 11). An Ayurvedic Approach to Anxiety. *Chopra.* https://chopra.com/articles/an-ayurvedic-approach-to-anxiety

Chibanda, D., Weiss, H. A., Verhey, R., Simms, V., Munjoma, R., Rusakaniko, S., ... & Araya, R. (2016). Effect of a primary care-based psychological intervention on symptoms of common mental disorders in Zimbabwe: A randomized clinical trial. *JAMA, 316*(24), 2618-2626.

Clemens, A. (2023). *The Mediating Effect of FOMO on the Relationship Between Social Media Engagement and Anxiety in College Students.* **Bridges: A Journal of Student Research,** 12(12), Article 3. Coastal Carolina University. Retrieved from https://digitalcommons.coastal.edu/bridges/vol12/iss12/3/

Chopra, D. (2005). *Peace is the Way: Bringing War and Violence to an End.* New York: Harmony Books.

Cohen, S., Janicki-Deverts, D., & Miller, G. E. (2016). Psychological stress and disease. *JAMA, 298*(14), 1685–1687. https://doi.org/10.1001/jama.298.14.1685

Craske, M. G., & Mystkowski, J. L. (2006). Exposure therapy and extinction: Clinical studies. *Anxiety, Stress & Coping, 19*(3), 251–272.

Cromie, W. J. (2002). Treating ills with music: From anxiety to Alzheimer's, from pain to Parkinson's. *Harvard University Gazette Staff.*

Cuijpers, P., & Smit, F. (2004). Subthreshold depression as a risk indicator for major depressive disorder: A systematic review of prospective studies. *Acta Psychiatrica Scandinavica, 109*(5), 325–331.

Cyberpsychology, Behavior, and Social Networking. (May 2022). Taking a one-week break from social media improves well-being, depression, and anxiety: A randomized controlled trial. Retrieved from https://www.liebertpub.com/doi/10.1089/cyber.2021.0324

Diego, M. A., Jones, N. A., & Field, T. (1998). Aromatherapy positively affects mood, EEG patterns of alertness, and math computations. *International Journal of Neuroscience, 96*(3-4), 217-224.

Drake, K. (2022). Biofeedback for anxiety: How it works. *Psych Central.* Retrieved from https://psychcentral.com/anxiety/managing-anxiety-with-biofeedback

Epstein, M., & Miller, M. V. Buddhist therapy. Seminar conducted at The Tibet House, New York City.

Essential Science Publishing. (2004). *Essential Oils Desk Reference* (3rd ed.).

Evans-Lacko, S., London, J., Little, K., Henderson, C., & Thornicroft, G. (2013). Evaluation of a brief anti-stigma campaign in Cambridge: Do short-term campaigns work? *BMC Public Health, 10*(13), 495.

Field, T., Ironson, G., Scafidi, F., Nawrocki, T., Goncalves, A., Burman, I., Pickens, J., Fox, N., Schanberg, S., & Kuhn, C. (1996). Massage therapy reduces anxiety and enhances EEG pattern of alertness and math computations. *International Journal of Neuroscience, 86*(3-4), 197-205.

Ford, D. E., & Kamerow, D. B. (1989). Epidemiologic study of sleep disturbances and psychiatric disorders: An opportunity for prevention? *JAMA, 262*(11), 1479-1484.

Foster, S. (1996). *Herbs for Your Health.* Loveland, CO: Interweave Press.

Friedman, J. (2005). *Earth's Elders: The Wisdom of The World's Oldest People.* South Kent, CT: Earth's Elders Foundation.

Hay, L. L. (1987). *You Can Heal Your Life.* Santa Monica, CA: Hay House.

Hayes, S. C., Strosahl, K. D., & Wilson, K. G. (2003). *Acceptance and Commitment Therapy: An Experiential Approach to Behavior Change.* Guilford Press.

Hayes, S. C., Luoma, J. B., Bond, F. W., Masuda, A., & Lillis, J. (2006). Acceptance and commitment therapy: Model, processes, and outcomes. *Behaviour Research and Therapy, 44*(1), 1-25.

Mindful. (2019, June 12). How to meditate for anxiety. Retrieved from https://www.mindful.org/mindfulness-meditation-anxiety

Hofmann, S. G., Sawyer, A. T., Witt, A. A., & Oh, D. (2010). The effect of mindfulness-based therapy on anxiety and depression: A meta-analytic review. *Journal of Consulting and Clinical Psychology, 78*(2), 169–183.

Hofmann, S. G., Asnaani, A., Vonk, I. J. J., Sawyer, A. T., & Fang, A. (2012). The efficacy of cognitive behavioral therapy: A review of meta-analyses. *Cognitive Therapy and Research, 36*(5), 427–440.

Hunt, M. G., Marx, R., Lipson, C., & Young, J. (2018). No more FOMO: Limiting social media decreases loneliness and depression. *Journal of Social and Clinical Psychology, 37*(10), 751-768.

Hyman, M. (2009). *The Ultra Mind Solution.* New York, NY: Scribner.

House, J. S., et al. (1988). Social relationships and health. *Science, 241,* 540–545. https://doi.org/10.1126/science.3399889

Janis, S. (2008). *Spirituality for Dummies.* Hoboken, NJ: Wiley Publishing Inc.

Johnson, B., et al. (20YY). Music therapy for generalized anxiety disorder: A randomized controlled trial. *Journal of Music Therapy.*

Journal of Psychosomatic Research. (1989). Vol. 23, Issue 2, 197-206.

Kashdan, T. B., & Rottenberg, J. (2010). Psychological flexibility as a fundamental aspect of health. *Clinical Psychology Review, 30*(7), 865-878.

Kawachi, I., & Berkman, L. F. (2001). Social ties and mental health. *Journal of Urban Health, 78*(3), 458-467.

Kasper, S., Müller, W. E., Volz, H. P., Möller, H. J., Koch, E., & Dienel, A. (2018). Silexan in anxiety disorders: Clinical data and pharmacological background. *World Journal of Biological Psychiatry, 19*(6), 412-420.

Kennedy, R. (2024). *Anxiety Rx: A Revolutionary Prescription for Anxiety Relief—from the Doctor Who Created It.* St. Martin's Essentials.

Kerslake, R. (2021). How cognitive behavioral therapy can treat your anxiety. *Healthline*. Retrieved from https://www.healthline.com/health/anxiety/cbt-for-anxiety

Keville, K., & Green, M. *Aromatherapy: A Complete Guide to the Healing Art*. Freedom, CA: Crossing Press.

Kohnen, R. O. (1988). The effects of valerian, propranolol, and their combination on activation performance and mood of healthy volunteers under social stress conditions. *Pharmacopsychiatry, 21*, 447-448.

Kozasa, E. H., Santos, R. F., Rueda, A. D., Benedito-Silva, A. A., De Ornellas, F. L., & Leite, J. R. (2008). Evaluation of Siddha Samadhi Yoga for anxiety and depression symptoms: A preliminary study. Research study at the Universidade Federal de Sao Paulo.

Kliger, B., & Lee, R. (2004). *Integrative Medicine: Principles for Practice*. New York, NY: McGraw-Hill.

Léger, D., & Bayon, V. (2010). Societal costs of insomnia. *Sleep Medicine Reviews, 14*(6), 379-389.

Li, Y., Li, Y., Winkelman, J. W., et al. (2021). Insomnia and risk of future depression and anxiety in adults. *Journal of Clinical Sleep Medicine, 17*(4), 643-651.

Lu, G., Jia, R., Liang, D., Yu, J., Wu, Z., & Chen, C. (2021). Effects of music therapy on anxiety: A meta-analysis of randomized controlled trials. *Psychiatry Research, 304*, 114137.

Maté, Gabor. *When the Body Says No: Exploring the Stress-Disease Connection*. John Wiley & Sons, 2003.

Maté, Gabor. *The Myth of Normal: Depression, Anxiety, and the Human Cost of Stress*. Avery, 2023.

Mayo Clinic. Retrieved from https://www.mayoclinic.com

Mel Robbins Podcast. (2024). *The Toolkit for Healing Anxiety, Part 2* [Podcast episode featuring Dr. Russell Kennedy]. Retrieved from https://www.melrobbins.com/episode/episode-57

Meshi, D., Morawetz, C., & Heekeren, H. R. (2019). Nucleus accumbens response to gains in reputation for the self relative to gains for others predicts social media use. *Journal of Computer-Mediated Communication, 24*(3), 124-138.

Mennini, T., Bernasconi, P., & Bombardelli, E. (1993). In vitro study on the interaction of extracts and pure compounds from *Valeriana officinalis* roots with GABA, benzodiazepine, and barbiturate receptors. *Fitoterapia, 64*, 291-300.

Mitchell, A. J., et al. (2023). *Understanding the Relationship Between Smartphone Use and Anxiety in University Students: A Qualitative Study*. **JMIR Formative Research,** 7, e43037. Retrieved from https://formative.jmir.org/2023/1/e43037

Morarend, Q., & Andrews, S. R. (2019). Biofeedback and relaxation techniques. In *StatPearls [Internet]*. StatPearls Publishing.

Motomura, N., Sakurai, A., & Yotsuya, Y. (2001). Reduction of mental stress with lavender odorant. *Perceptual and Motor Skills, 93*(3), 713-718.

Murray, M., Pizzorno, J., & Pizzorno, L. (2005). *Encyclopedia of Healing Foods*. New York, NY: Atria Books.

Naslund, J. A., Grande, S. W., Aschbrenner, K. A., & Elwyn, G. (2016). Naturally occurring peer support through social media: The experiences of individuals with severe mental illness using YouTube. *PloS One, 9*(10), e110171.

Nagalingam, A., et al. *"Probiotic supplementation and anxiety: A systematic review and meta-analysis of randomized controlled trials"* (2020)

Neustadt, J. (2007). *A Revolution in Health Through Nutritional Biochemistry.* iUniverse, Inc.

Ng, Q. X., Venkatanarayanan, N., & Loke, W. *"Gut microbiome composition and anxiety in humans: A systematic review"* (2020)

Nguyen, K. T., Hoang, H. T. X., Bui, Q. V., Chan, D. N. S., Choi, K. C., & Chan, C. W. H. (2023). Effects of music intervention combined with progressive muscle relaxation on anxiety, depression, stress, and quality of life among women with cancer receiving chemotherapy: A pilot randomized controlled trial. *PloS One, 18*(11), e0293060. https://doi.org/10.1371/journal.pone.0293060

Öst, L.-G. (2014). The efficacy of acceptance and commitment therapy: An updated systematic review and meta-analysis. *Behaviour Research and Therapy, 61*, 105-121.

Ohayon, M. M. (2002). Epidemiology of insomnia: What we know and what we still need to learn. *Sleep Medicine Reviews, 6*(2), 97-111. https://doi.org/10.1053/smrv.2001.0186

Pfeiffer, P. N., Heisler, M., Piette, J. D., Rogers, M. A., & Valenstein, M. (2011). Efficacy of peer support interventions for depression: A meta-analysis. *General Hospital Psychiatry, 33*(1), 29-36.

Pratte, M. A., Nanavati, K. B., Young, V., & Morley, C. P. (2014). An alternative treatment for anxiety: A systematic review of human trial results reported for the Ayurvedic herb ashwagandha *(Withania somnifera). Journal of Alternative and Complementary Medicine, 20*(12), 901-908. https://doi.org/10.1089/acm.2014.0177

Prutt, G. (2022). *EFT Tapping for Anxiety | The Recovery Village.* Retrieved from https://www.therecoveryvillage.com/mental-health/anxiety/eft-tapping/

Przybylski, A. K., Murayama, K., DeHaan, C. R., & Gladwell, V. (2013). Motivational, emotional, and behavioral correlates.

Rothschild, D. *Psychologist Interview.* New York.

Shapiro, P. *Licensed Acupuncturist and Herbalist Interview.* New York.

Smith, A., et al. (2021). The impact of music therapy on anxiety: A meta-analysis. Journal of Clinical Psychology.

Southwick, S. M., Litz, B. T., Charney, D., & Friedman, M. J. (2011). *Resilience and Mental Health: Challenges Across the Lifespan.* Cambridge University Press.

Stabler, C. (2021). *The Effects of Social Media on Mental Health.* Retrieved from https://www.lancastergeneralhealth.org/health-hub-home/2021/september/the-effects-of-social-media-on-mental-health

Thoits, P. A. (2011). Mechanisms linking social ties and support to physical and mental health. *Journal of Health and Social Behavior, 52*(2), 145-161.

Tifferet, S., & Vilnai-Yavetz, I. (2017). 'I like therefore I am': The association between Facebook use and self-esteem in women and men. *New Media & Society, 19*(3), 357-376.

Tolle, E. (2005). *A New Earth: Awakening to Your Life's Purpose.* New York, NY: Dutton/Penguin Group.

Tyler, V. E. (1981). *The Honest Herbal: A Sensible Guide to the Use of Herbs and Related Remedies.* Philadelphia, PA: G.F. Stickley Co.

University of Texas. (2006). *Anxiety and Depression.* Retrieved from http://www.johnshopkinshealthalerts.com/alerts/depression_anxiety/JohnsHopkinsHealthAlertsDepressionAnxiety_1492-1.html

Vogel, E. A., Rose, J. P., Okdie, B. M., Eckles, K., & Franz, B. (2018). Who compares and despairs? The effect of social comparison orientation on social media use and its outcomes. *Journal of Social and Clinical Psychology, 37*(9), 751-768.

Vosoughi, S., Roy, D., & Aral, S. (2018). The spread of true and false news online. *Science, 359*(6380), 1146-1151.

Waelder, L. C., Uddo, M., Marquett, R., Ropelato, M., Freightman, S., Pardo, A., & Salazer, J. (2008). *Pilot Study of Meditation on Mental Health Workers Following Hurricane Katrina.* Research study by Pacific Graduate Institute of Psychology. Retrieved abstract from PUBMED.

Walach, H., Rilling, C., & Engelke, U. (1999). *International Society of Technology Assessment in Health Care Meeting.* University of Freiburg, Department of Psychology, Freiburg, Germany.

Walsh, D. (2022). *Social Media Use Linked To A Decline In Mental Health.* Retrieved from https://mitsloan.mit.edu/ideas-made-to-matter/study-social-media-use-linked-to-decline-mental-health

Watson, K. (2018). *Can Acupuncture Help with Anxiety?* Retrieved from https://www.healthline.com/health/acupuncture-for-anxiety

Wilson, D. R. (2022). *Gut Health and Anxiety: Link and Ways to Manage.* Retrieved from https://www.medicalnewstoday.com/articles/gut-health-and-anxiety

Windle, G., Hughes, D., Linck, P., Russell, I., & Woods, R. T. (2011). Is exercise effective in promoting mental well-being in older age? A systematic review. *Aging & Mental Health, 14*(6), 652-669.

Winston, M. (2007). *Adaptogens.* Rochester, VT: Healing Arts Press.

Wong, A. H. C. (2000). Herbal remedies in psychiatric practice. In P. B. Fontanarosa (Ed.), *Alternative Medicine: An Objective Assessment* (pp. 386–401). Chicago: American Medical Association.

World Health Organization. (2007). *Assessment of the Risk of Hepatotoxicity With Kava Products.*

Worwood, Valerie Ann. (1991). *The Complete Book of Essential Oils and Aromatherapy.* San Rafael, CA: New World Library.

Resources and Suggested Further Reading on CBD

The Big Book of Terps – Understanding Terpenes, Flavonoids, & Synergy in Cannabis by Russ Hudson. https://www.thebigbookofterps.com

LabCBD and LabCannamist Certification Course Material by Colleen Quinn. https://www.labaroma.com/certified-courses

The CBD Oil Miracle by Laura Lagano, MS, RDN, CDN

Leaf411.org Hotline run by cannabis nurses

Taming THC: Potential Cannabis Synergy and Phytocannabinoid-Terpenoid Entourage Effects by Ethan B. Russo. *British Journal of Pharmacology.* https://www.ncbi.nlm.nih.gov/pmc/articles/PMC3165946/

Neural Basis of Anxiolytic Effects of Cannabidiol (CBD) in Generalized Social Anxiety Disorder: A Preliminary Report by J. Crippa, G. N. Derenusson. *Journal of Psychopharmacology.* https://www.semanticscholar.org/paper/Neural-basis-of-anxiolytic-effects-of-cannabidiol-a-Crippa-Derenusson/b57ecc86be5d21fabd6ce116a8d7c34b4ff4b337

The Endocannabinoid System: Essential and Mysterious by Peter Grinspoon, MD. *Harvard Health Publishing.* https://www.health.harvard.edu/blog/the-endocannabinoid-system-essential-and-mysterious-202108112569

Resources

Acupuncture
http://www.nccaom.org

Aromatherapy Essential Oils
https://enfleurage.com
http://www.naturesgift.com
http://mountainroseherbs.com

Bach Flower Essences
http://www.bachflower.com

Biofeedback
http://www.bcia.org

CBD
www.rosebudcbd.com
www.shop-poplar.com (LabCannamist brand)
www.bloomfarmscbd.com
www.charlottesweb.com
www.blacktiecbd.net

Cognitive Behavioral Therapy
http://www.nacbt.org

Eye Movement Desensitization and Reprocessing (EMDR)
https://www.emdr.com

Homeopathy
Go to the services section of the website below to find a homeopathic practitioner

http://nationalcenterforhomeopathy.org

Music Therapy
http://www.musictherapy.org

Reiki
http://www.reiki.org

Reflexology
http://www.reflexology-usa.org

www.ingramcontent.com/pod-product-compliance
Lightning Source LLC
Chambersburg PA
CBHW070635030426
42337CB00020B/4020